the P☀sitive Birth Book

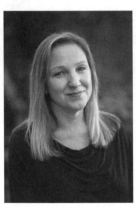

photo Bill Bradshaw

About the author

Milli Hill is a writer who lives in Somerset with her partner and three small children. In 2012 she set up The Positive Birth Movement (PBM), a global network of antenatal discussion groups, with the aim of improving childbirth and giving women better access to support and information, not anticipating the huge appetite among women for more positive messages about birth. What started as a small idea became a global phenomenon, with over 400 groups around the world.

As well as running the PBM, Milli also writes for various publications about all things birth, breastfeeding and motherhood. For over two years she wrote a popular column for *Best magazine*, and she's now a columnist for *Telegraph Women*.

the Positive Birth Book

A new approach to pregnancy, birth and the early weeks

by Milli Hill

pinter & martin

For George

Disclaimer: Please note that this book provides general information about pregnancy, labour and birth and does not constitute medical advice for individuals. Please consult your own healthcare providers when making decisions that may affect your health or that of your baby: throughout the book you will find suggestions about how to communicate your wishes clearly and work with the professionals involved in your care. If you need further support or advice please see the resources section at the back of the book for links to organisations that may be able to help.

The Positive Birth Book: A new approach to pregnancy, birth and the early weeks
First published by Pinter & Martin Ltd 2017, reprinted 2017
© 2017 Milli Hill
Illustrations Kate Evans
Milli Hill has asserted her moral right to be identified as the author of this work in accordance with the Copyright, Designs and Patents Act of 1988.

ISBN 978-1-78066-430-9

Also available as ebook

British Library Cataloguing-in-Publication Data
A catalogue record for this book is available from the British Library.

Editor Susan Last
Index by Helen Bilton
Proofread by Debbie Kennett

Set in LinoLetter

Printed and bound in the UK by Ashford Colour Press

Pinter & Martin Ltd
6 Effra Parade
London SW2 1PS

www.pinterandmartin.com

Contents

❦ Introduction ❧

What kind of birth do you really want? Sometimes it's difficult to answer that question really honestly, and it can feel so overwhelming that it's tempting to do the well-known Ostrich Manoeuvre. This book wants to encourage you to keep your head well away from the sand and really focus on planning and preparing for the best birth possible. It doesn't want you to 'go with the flow', or feel that it's selfish to worry about your own experience of childbirth because 'all that matters is a healthy baby'.

This book is here to tell you that you matter too. Yes, it goes without saying that a healthy baby is the number one goal of childbirth, and *The Positive Birth Book* doesn't want to challenge that, but it does want to get a red pen out and remove 'healthy baby' from its current status as 'pinnacle of expectations' and demote it to 'baseline'.

You matter. Wanting to have a brilliant birth experience is not selfish. When a child is born, as they say, so is a mother, and motherhood, as you are perhaps about to discover, requires you to be strong, tough, mentally and physically healthy, happy, and madly in love with your children. What better way to set this all in motion than with a truly positive birth?

In today's culture, birth is in crisis. Television shows paint a bleak picture of women struggling and suffering on their backs, caesarean rates are at an all time high of over 25 per cent, and many mums-to-be – and dads-to-be too – are scared or even dreading the event. But the truth is, while birth on TV may look like a frightening medical procedure, it doesn't have to be this way. Birth can be a very beautiful thing: the perfect expression of your female body at its healthiest and most vital.

Many of the simple ingredients to make birth positive have been forgotten. For starters, we are mammals – and what self-respecting cat or dog do you know who would give birth effectively in a brightly lit room, with a stranger leaning on their leg and casually chatting to their husband about the footie scores? To have the best chance of a normal birth, we need to get back to basics: darkness, stillness, familiarity – and this book will show you how, regardless of whether you choose home, birth centre or hospital.

How we give birth matters – and not just for the day itself. An empowering, confident start can have a lifelong impact on the physical and emotional health of both mum and baby. From the importance of early attachment and bonding, to emerging evidence on the vital role birth plays in the human microbiome, this book stresses the far-reaching value of a normal, natural birth.

But don't feel this book is only for you if you want a candlelit home birth with crocheted bunting. Positive birth is about having freedom of choice, access to accurate information, and feeling in control, powerful and respected. If, for you, this means choosing an epidural or an elective caesarean, then this book will help you to make that choice with confidence and have the birth that feels exactly right for you on the day. It will also equip you to deal with inevitable wild cards and stay in control of your choices no matter how birth unfolds.

The Positive Birth Book urges women to wake up from the twilight sleep of the highly medicalised 1960s and 70s and demand more information, more options and more respect in the birth room. For some reason, 21st-century women who are happy to stand up for their rights in the board room or the bedroom are still taking childbirth lying down. Many birth stories still contain the phrase 'They let me' or 'I was not allowed'. This book will give you the confidence to stand up for the birth you want and learn about your rights and choices. Yes – you have rights and choices!

This is the key to a positive birth. Knowing that your birth really matters, and feeling at all times that you have rights and choices, and that you are being fully consulted and listened to, will make all the difference to your experience. I want to tell you everything I've learned, not just from years of reading, writing and talking about childbirth, but from my own journey as a mother of three. I hope this book helps you to understand the true meaning of positive birth, to feel confident in the possibility that birth will be the best moment of your life, and to anticipate the big day with a lot less fear and a whole heap more eye-sparkling excitement.

My birth stories

I can still remember the moments that followed my first positive pregnancy test. Alone in the house, I stood in front of the long bathroom mirror. Contemplating my reflection, I had two clear thoughts.

Thought 1: Oh. My. God. There's a BABY in there.
Thought 2: Oh. My. GOD!! It's got to get OUT!

The rest of my very long pregnancy was largely spent preoccupied with these two thoughts, mostly the second one. I was 31, in love with my partner, and thrilled to be expecting. At the same time, I also felt like someone who had got drunk and agreed to do a parachute jump, only to find when they sobered up that backing out simply wasn't an option, and that – worse still – the plane had already left the ground.

For the entire pregnancy, I felt like I was several thousand feet up and about to freefall against my will. I cried uncontrollably at the slightest opportunity, which, as women often do, I blamed on 'hormones'. But actually, I was just bloody terrified. They were 'tears for fears'.

It's well known that there are two basic responses to human fear: fight or flight. In pregnancy, so often a time of great fear for women, this can translate into taking one of two paths – neither of which is 'right' or 'wrong'. Some women go for 'flight' and just don't engage with the situation. They use phrases like, 'I'm just going to go with the flow', or, 'There's no point preparing for birth because it's so unpredictable'. Then there are the 'fight' group, who turn having a baby into a PhD. I fell into the latter category.

I read every book I could get my hands on, even a history of birth. I attended several courses, both on my own and with my partner. I joined online groups and I googled things. A lot. Often in the middle of the night. I planned a home birth on the advice of two different friends, both midwives, who told me I'd be less likely to have interventions and added, 'At home you get two midwives. In hospital you're lucky if you get one'.

As I got nearer to the big day, things started to get political. Suddenly my midwives, who had been all smiles about my birth plans up to that point, told me that I might not be able to have my baby at home after all. 'If there aren't enough of us on duty when you go into labour, you'll just have to come in to hospital.' The obligatory google revealed that this was a common story – almost every woman who was planning a home birth was getting this late memo.

Conspiracy theories abounded. 'They wait until you are too pregnant to argue before they give you the bad news', was a common theme, and most home birth websites and groups told stories of women 'standing their ground', even in the throes of labour, and engaging in a kind of Mexican stand-off with the midwives, in which a baby slipping out on the bathroom floor with no professionals to catch it became the ultimate bullet.

This did not help with my already sky-high terror levels.

However, I channelled my hormonal rage and fired off letters to my MP and Head of Midwifery. This did little to help, but it did at least give me a project for the strange couple of weeks of maternity leave before the baby was born, and it was arguably more stimulating than picking out nursery colour schemes.

What happened next would make my home birth crusade pale into a distant memory. My due date arrived: 21 December. I went to a festive party that night and took great pleasure in answering the inevitable question, 'When are you due?' by saying brightly 'Today!'. This seemed to scare the life out of people, who were perhaps expecting an *Eastenders*-style delivery in which I gave birth under the Christmas tree without even having time to remove my tights.

Sadly, perhaps, there was no such drama. The days passed, and Christmas was tense. The comical reindeer babygro we had hoped to dress our newborn in was put aside, and everything in general became a lot less funny. The phone rang just after Christmas. It was the hospital, and I was summoned to see a consultant. 'Uh-oh', my wry midwife friend told me. 'You're becoming a problem. They've decided to get a man in.'

She was right. After months of midwife-led care, I found myself in the office of a very big bloke in a suit. I was a week 'overdue'. He told me that the risk of stillbirth would increase if I went past 42 weeks and said that he wanted to book me in to be induced in a few days' time. He also offered to give me a 'sweep'. (See page 224. He had very big fingers. I declined.)

I had four sweeps done by the midwives who continued to visit me at home, and in spite of extreme needle phobia I tried daily acupuncture. As things got more desperate, I went for bumpy car rides, ate multiple pineapples, meditated, visualised and chanted. Finally, at 42 weeks, I drank castor oil, which, for those of you who are curious, tastes like melted tea-lights and makes you shit through the eye of a needle. If you're still curious (and I'd understand if that last piece of information had dampened your appetite slightly), turn to page 223 to read about natural induction.

The castor oil did seem to have some kind of effect, other than that described above. A trip into hospital for monitoring confirmed I was having very mild contractions, visible on the graph and regular. 'Go home and have your baby', they said. 'But before you leave, let's just give you one more really *vigorous* sweep.'

World-renowned midwife Ina May Gaskin (see page 169) would have been horrified by this suggestion. The cervix, she explains, is a sphincter muscle, and like all other sphincter muscles, it will completely close for business if it doesn't feel comfortable and safe. And this, I believe, is what happened to me. My shy little cervix, which was presumably just beginning to get going on Project Labour, didn't like that vigorous sweep one bit. It slammed shut in horror – and those mild contractions in hospital were the last signs of natural labour I experienced. A few days later, at 42+3, I agreed to be induced.

They say what doesn't kill you makes you stronger and it's certainly true that all of my experiences played a huge part in shaping the passion for improving childbirth that I have today. My induction ended in a healthy baby, my completely beautiful and loved little girl, Bess. But it also ended with my feet in stirrups, an episiotomy, and a forceps delivery. It ended in an unpleasant third stage in which the obstetrician leaned on my stomach in a way that made me feel hugely embarrassed and objectified. And it ended in several months of struggling to come to terms with some of my birth memories, as I felt shattered and more than a little bit lost.

From personal experience I learnt how hurtful it can be to be told that 'you have a healthy baby and that is all that matters'. My experience set in motion many thoughts about what needed to change about birth so that as few women as possible would start motherhood feeling physically and emotionally damaged. But changing birth for everyone else would have to wait: first, I had to change it for myself.

My second daughter was born at home in a birth pool, with her dad, two midwives, her auntie and her two-year-old sister present. I had asked the midwives in panic during that pregnancy, 'But what shall I do with my toddler! Surely she can't be around at the time of the birth?!'. 'Why not?', they asked me. 'What don't you want her to see?'

Their question challenged me, and revealed to me just how much I was still misinformed about childbirth. With their help, I was able to reframe my perception, and to anticipate birth as something calm, normal and beautiful. There would be no screaming, no bloodbath, no loss of dignity, no begging for drugs. All the things I had been told about birth as I grew up as a woman in 20th-century Western culture, I needed to unlearn.

Finally, I did something that I had been too scared to do in my first pregnancy. I watched birth films. I can still remember the one that affected me most: in a darkened room, a woman was on all fours in a birth pool. There was no sound but the gentle lapping of water as her body made small rocking motions back and forth. Every few minutes, she made what could only be described as a low mooing sound. Then, with a sudden movement upwards that broke the sense of tranquillity, she reached down and in a few splashing motions brought her baby to the water's surface.

I was transfixed. This did not look scary at all. It was so peaceful, so everyday. And nobody touched her, nobody 'egged her on' with incessant chants of 'push'; nobody took her baby, declared its sex or wiped it or cut its cord.

This was the birth I aimed for, and although it wasn't quite like this, it came close. I still had so many fears, and, although I was already a mother, I felt in some ways a novice: I'd never gone into labour naturally, and I'd never pushed a baby out unaided, for starters. So I panicked a bit, and cried a bit, and doubted myself quite a lot. I didn't quite have the confidence of the quiet moo-er in the dark pool – I was a bit more flappy and a bit more vocal. But in the end, my 10lb 4oz daughter came out quickly and easily, with only a small tear that did not need stitching.

I had independent midwives (IMs). I always feel slightly awkward about confessing to this, as I'm aware that many people are not able to afford to 'go private'. What prompted my choice was finding out that my local NHS midwives were now operating on a 'bank' system, making it likely, they told me, that I would a) not know my midwife and b) get a midwife who had never attended a home birth, let alone a water birth. There was still the problem of them potentially not being able to attend at all due to staff shortages. I lost confidence in the system, and got my chequebook out.

Of all the financial decisions I've made in my life – many of which have been really rubbish – this must be the one I'm most at ease with. For the amazing, loving and supportive care that I received, and the blissful, joyful birth experience that ensued, I would have paid much, much more. Many people dig deep in their pockets or get help from family to make their wedding day really special. Why should the day we have our babies be any different?

Giving birth 'outside the system' suited me well because my body clearly did not want to fit in with the system. Again I went 'overdue', but this time I just sat it out, with no sweeps, pineapples or other desperate measures. My baby came at 42 weeks on the dot. Had I been under NHS care, I would almost certainly have been induced again.

My independent midwives exuded confidence in women's bodies and this enabled them to stand back and trust me to be the ultimate decision-maker. This kind of care should be available to all women, not just the lucky few. After that great home water birth experience I set up the Positive Birth Movement (PBM), in the hopes that by creating a network of groups where women could come together and share information and stories, birth could change for the better. Often 'the system' gets the rap for women's negative birth experiences, but maybe if women – who are, after all, 'the consumers' – had a better awareness of their choices and rights, they would become more demanding, and the system would have no choice but to accommodate them.

The PBM – which started as just a small idea – spread like wildfire. Within just a few weeks there were groups popping up all over the UK and beyond, and at the time of writing we have nearly 450 groups spread all across the globe.

> **Positive Birth is defined by the following criteria:**
>
> **1** Women are where they want to be
>
> **2** Choices are informed by reality not fear
>
> **3** Women are listened to and treated with respect and dignity
>
> **4** Mothers are empowered and enriched
>
> **5** Memories are warm and proud

This definition really resonates with people, and cuts through the polarised representation of birthing women – 'too posh to push' versus 'hairy homebirthers' – allowing women to decide for themselves what positive birth means to them. Through the PBM I have discovered just what a huge appetite women have for more positive information about what birth is really like, and how relieved they are when they are given a chance to replace their fears with facts.

When I gave birth to my third – and final – baby, I was a long way from the terrified girl in the mirror who had stared at her reflection like a rabbit in the headlights. I wasn't terrified any more, and I knew I could do it. That isn't to say that I 'birthed without fear' – I personally think it is normal to have some 'fear' of giving birth – if by fear we mean a healthy respect for the enormity of a particular event. I planned another home birth, but was well aware that just because I had had one blissful and smooth experience, it didn't mean that I was automatically entitled to another one.

I was also pretty worried that I was growing another whopper, and, in the wee small hours that most pregnant women are familiar with, I would lie awake sometimes and imagine a hospital transfer and a caesarean for my enormous baby. Again, I went past my due date. Again, I told my midwife I wished to 'do nothing' (see page 225), and she respected my choice.

My little boy was born at precisely 42 weeks after a calm and magical night spent in the birth pool, listening to favourite music and riding the contractions as they intensified. The experience was a glorious mix of every emotion you could name, and there were moments when I felt like a goddess, and moments when I felt like it was the worst thing that had ever happened to me, and everything in between. He was 9 pounds 11 (4.4 kg): his sister is still proud that she kept her title of my 'biggest baby', and prouder still that she was the one to cut his cord.

This book is not my attempt to convince you to have home births, as I did. Nor do I want to suggest you decline all intervention or go to war with your care providers. You can have the most brilliant birth after a hospital induction; you can have the most fantastic elective caesarean; you can have an epidural and still be the goddess you deserve to be. The key is not in the choices you make, but in feeling at all times that you *have* choices. This flows as a natural consequence from being informed, and understanding your rights.

And so I reach out of the pages of this book, and offer you a tandem skydive. I was that terrified girl in the mirror once, and I know how it feels to be 10,000 feet up and all out of options. But birth must happen, so let's make it the ride of your life. We are strapped together, the parachute is on my back, my hand is on the rip-cord. Let's jump!

Chapter 1

What do you bring to birth?

In birth preparation, this question is often phrased the other way around. What will birth bring to me? What will my birth be like? What will I do if this happens, or that? These questions are important, but before we ask them, we need to look at the situation a little more deeply, and consider that who we are, and how we feel about birth, can and will have an impact on how our birth experience unfolds.

We all think we know a little bit about what birth is like, even if we are pregnant for the first time. But where did that information come from? Most likely the answer is family, and the wider culture such as television and the media. We might have been told something about how we ourselves were born, or seen women in labour on our favourite soap. Maybe we overheard a hushed conversation between grown-ups when we were children, or perhaps we were shown a film of birth in school.

Whatever the source, we need to question it now. It's really important to carefully unpack the 'baggage' that we might be bringing with us into our own labours, and ask some vital questions: what am I expecting birth to be like? Where do I get these expectations from and are they the true picture? And how might my expectations of birth affect my reality?

The broken chain of wisdom

Up until fairly recently in western women's history, birth took place in the community, and was therefore more visible, and probably more audible, than it is today. Women did not disappear to the hospital and return with a newborn. The sights and sounds of birth would have been part of the fabric of life, a domestic affair that family, neighbours and friends were all involved in.

Fast-forward to the medicalised births of the past few decades. For all the advantages that modern medicine brings, there's no denying that there have been some hospital practices that have been to the detriment of women: the pubic shave, the enema, the routine use of stirrups and episiotomies, to name just a few. In the hospital births of the 1960s, 70s and beyond, women became quite passive in the experience – having a baby was something that was done 'to them' rather than 'by them', and consent was not often sought. Babies were whisked away to nurseries, and if anyone 'owned' birth at this time, it was the stern Matron of the ward, rather than the mother herself.

When it comes to childbearing, we are the 'three monkeys generation': we have not seen birth, have not heard birth, and have not been spoken to about birth. Our mothers, and for some of us, our grandmothers, often gave birth under disempowering circumstances they would rather forget. Birth, if it is talked about, is often described as a time when you will have to 'leave your dignity at the door', and suffer the worst pain you can imagine. There are rarely any positive messages. Is it any wonder we are all terrified?

This broken chain of wisdom affects breastfeeding too. Many of us were formula fed ourselves and have never seen anybody breastfeed. The effect that this interruption to intergenerational knowledge has on our confidence in our bodies' abilities to birth and feed our babies cannot be underestimated.

※ What messages about birth have you been given by your closest family?

※ What have you been told about your own birth?

※ Are the words and stories you have heard positive, or negative?

※ How do they make you feel about your own forthcoming birth experience?

School education

Many of us were taught about childbirth at school and some of us were shown still pictures or films of birth to support this learning. Unfortunately, these films and images were often 'of the age': women lying on a bed, on their back, looking pretty terrified and helpless. Perhaps, either intentionally or unintentionally, they served the purpose of deterring young girls from pregnancy. Whatever the motivation, many of these films did (and sadly often still do) a great job of instilling a fear of birth in a whole generation of women.

> ☀ Did you see images or films of birth when you were at school?
>
> ☀ What message do you think these films gave you about what birth would be like?
>
> ☀ What was the teacher like and what might his or her own experiences of birth have been?

Birth on TV

Think about it. You want to make an advert that shows a young couple getting into the car on their way to hospital. The woman is in labour. How can you get this across to your viewer? Well, she has to look a certain way, of course. She has to look worried, in pain, and she's usually leaning weakly on her husband and seemingly unable to walk unaided. Of course, women in labour don't often actually look like this, but if you showed her striding to the car, eating a hot dog and shouting, 'Don't forget the bag you wazzock', to her partner, the viewer might not get the message.

Advertising, soap operas and TV dramas all follow the same format. 'Woman in labour' is a stock image that actresses must faithfully portray, and it usually includes weakness, distress, panic, and submission to the direction of those around her, be they 18th-century doctors, Colin Firth and Patrick Dempsey, or the entire cast of the soap telling her to, 'Push!' on the floor of the pub toilets.

Then we have the 'real life' dramas; the fly-on-the-wall

documentaries. Surely they show us what birth is really like?

Not quite. For starters, they are heavily edited to make the programme fast-paced and interesting. A long labour where mum potters about in the garden, has a snooze and makes a few phone calls might be lovely, but is unlikely to hold the viewer's attention. Secondly, these programmes often show very medicalised birth experiences. Inductions, for example, are great news for the producers, who can neatly schedule some easy daytime filming. And unfortunately, the births on these programmes are often – not always, but often – in a brightly lit, busy hospital room, with the woman on a bed, on her back.

As you'll discover as you read this book, this is one way to give birth, but it's certainly not the only way, and it's often associated with higher rates of intervention. As the saying goes, 'there's one born every minute', but I think most women would go off these programmes quite quickly if they realised how damaging this very one-sided portrayal of birth might be to their own experience.

☀ Do you watch birth documentaries?

☀ What kinds of births do you most often see on them?

☀ Have you ever seen an upright birth, a home birth, a birth centre birth, a water birth, or a woman-centred caesarean on a birth documentary?

☀ How do these types of shows make you feel about birth?

Birth – are you afraid?

The answer to this question is quite likely to be a big fat yes. You've only ever heard an eerie mix of horror stories and awkwardly loaded silence from friends and family on the subject, the film they showed you at school looked like a trip to the dentist that went horribly wrong, and every time you see a woman giving birth on TV she is screaming her head off and begging for it all to stop. Jovial phrases like, 'Pain worse than childbirth', and, 'Shitting a watermelon' don't do much to improve your confidence.

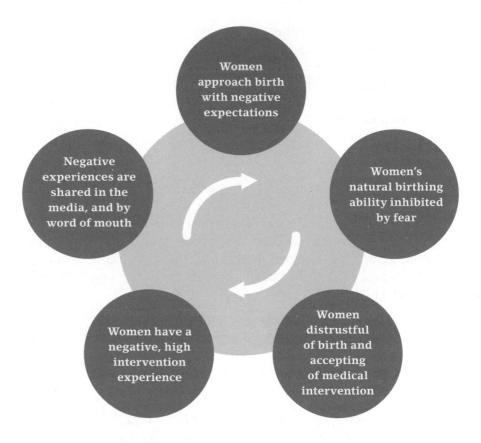

This fear – that most women feel – can have a direct impact on the kind of birth experience you end up having. First of all, it can make you less likely to research your options, less likely to assert your viewpoint or your rights, and more likely to decide to simply, 'lie back and think of England' – sometimes known as 'going with the flow'. Second, the expectation that birth is going to be extremely difficult and painful can cause high levels of adrenaline and physical tension in your body, which almost guarantees that your birth will be... you guessed it... extremely difficult and painful.

Expectations become reality, and fear becomes fact. After we have the dreadful birth we were completely expecting, we then have some really terrible stories to terrify other women with, and so the cycle continues.

The enemy of fear is information. The next chapter of this book will try to help you to challenge some of the negative expectations or assumptions you have built up over the course of your life about what giving birth will actually be like. If you are reading this during your pregnancy, it's possible that you will continue to get negative messages about birth from family, friends or even strangers, which may intensify as your pregnancy becomes more visible. They may ask, 'Have you decided what pain relief you're going to have?', or even humorously tease you, saying 'You'll never cope!'.

Imagine you were about to run a marathon, but that everyone you talked to about it looked worried and asked you, 'Are you sure you can do it?', 'I've heard the pain is terrible', or 'Did you know people sometimes die running marathons?'. Top athletes enlist the help of experts to ensure that their mind is entirely focused on the positive. They know how destructive thoughts can slow you down, and how powerful a confident mental attitude can be.

This is not an attempt to give you a false impression. Giving birth is tough, and yes, it is unpredictable. You might do loads of preparation for a home birth and then get pre-eclampsia and have your baby prematurely and on the operating table. You might plan a hospital birth with an epidural and have your baby at 3am on your living room floor. My least favourite 'birth affirmation' (see page 139) of all is: 'She believed she could so she did'. Telling women that if they just close their eyes and click their heels together hard enough, it will all go just how they want, is simply false.

But what we *can* do is maximise our chances. By challenging our preconceptions and our fears, by knowing our options and our rights, by understanding the optimal conditions for birth, and by making a clear plan for every eventuality, we can make getting the birth we want much more likely. So, now that we have begun to address some of the negative expectations you have of birth, our next step is to build up a more positive and accurate picture by asking: what is giving birth really like?

❧ Chapter 2 ❧

What is giving birth really like?

> 'Was childbirth painful for you?'
> 'No, no pain, but I know what the earth
> feels like making a mountain'.

This is the million dollar question for most pregnant women. It's great to challenge all your existing expectations of labour and birth, but, once you've done that, you need something concrete to replace them with. Of course, giving birth is as varied as there are women who do it. If we asked, 'What is making love really like?', or 'What is eating really like?', we wouldn't expect there to be one clear-cut, standard answer. Nevertheless, there is some common ground that most women share, so in this chapter we'll go through the process of a straightforward labour, bit by bit, hearing some juicy details from women who've been there and done that along the way. Then I'll try to answer some of the biggest questions about birth, including how much it hurts, and how much of a mess you're really going to make. Read on...

Labour in phases

There's a rather annoying tendency to break labour down into neat and tidy stages, and this comes from hospital birth, where

mathematical concepts like 'Friedman's curve', which measures
a woman's hourly rate of dilation, have been used for the past few
decades, both to assess the progress of labour, and to dictate when
there is not perceived to be enough progress and intervention is
necessary. In reality, most women's bodies don't conform to graphs,
charts and statistical norms – a labour may start slow, get fast, stall,
do a bit more slow stuff, then get cracking again, or it might be slow
all the way till the end, or it might be like riding the runaway horse
in the Derby.

You might hear in antenatal class about the 'Three Stages of
Labour'. This means the first phase of your uterus contracting
and your cervix dilating, the second phase, of being fully dilated
and pushing your baby out, and the third phase, often a bit of an
afterthought, of delivering the placenta.

Knowing about these three stages is useful, but it still doesn't
answer the question of how it all really feels. So let's look more
closely at what labour is like. I've divided it not into three phases,
but fourteen, although in reality all of these phases will blend and
blur into each other. Trying to conceptualise one of the most mind-
blowingly unique experiences of your life in this mathematical way
is a bit like trying to divide up your wedding day in terms of car
journeys, or measure out your life in coffee spoons.

It will be different for you. But it will also be something like this...

1. The Nothing Doing Phase

In the days and hours before labour begins, you might feel the
increasing intensity of the Nothing Doing Phase. You will be
desperately searching for signs that something is happening, and, in
particular if you are nearing your due date, you'll be being bombarded
by well-meaning friends asking, 'Anything doing?'

You might feel like the answer is, 'Nope, nothing to see here', but in
fact, the dance of hormones is almost certainly beginning, and there
may be internal changes that you cannot see or feel, like your baby
moving further into position or your cervix beginning to thin.

What does it feel like?

Boring, frustrating, exciting, heavy, cumbersome, and filled with
anticipation. Some women feel physically really uncomfortable, while
others are energised and agile. Many start to feel small urges to
withdraw from day-to-day life.

'I felt excited and full of bouncing energy one moment, withdrawn and reflective the next. Swinging emotions, spiralling thoughts – it was a roller coaster.' Olga Danyluk-Singh

'In those last few days I felt lost in a spiral of anticipation, pressure and impatience! I will always look back and wish I had been a little easier on myself in those magical last few moments. I'd have enjoyed looking at my body more, spent more time in the bath watching my bump ripple and made the most of alone time with my boyfriend.' Jen Muir

'I felt irritable, antsy. As if something was annoying me but I didn't know what.' Nyomi Winter

'Restless and in need of privacy in my nest.' Jay Kelly

'The last few days and hours are like constipation. You can feel it, you know it's there, you desperately want it to come out but it doesn't matter how hard you try, you know that bad boy isn't coming until it's good and ready. I hate constipation.' Suzy Ashworth

'So bored of waiting, impatient and yet for each subsequent pregnancy, I was more aware of what I was in for and tried to relish the final moments, the calm before the storm.' Wendy Evans

2. The Maybe Something is Happening Phase

This can sometimes be your mind playing tricks on you, due to your desperation to both meet your baby and be able to put on your own shoes again, but more often than not, it's the beginning of little signs that birth is more and more imminent. You might experience an increase in so-called 'Braxton Hicks', those tightenings in your bump that are like practice contractions. You might feel 'hormonal', perhaps with rushes of oxytocin, which can make you feel very positive and loved up, or adrenaline, which can make you decide that now would be a great time to launder your curtains by hand. You might also lose your mucus plug, which is the little blob of jelly that seals up your uterus. This will sometimes have a pinkish tinge and is also known rather romantically as a Bloody Show.

What does it feel like?

Spiralling inwards, feeling connected to your baby, nervous, excited, emotional, with some tightenings in your bump.

'This phase was funny for me. I was face timing my friend laughing thinking, "Is it or isn't it?!"' Lora Wilshaw

'I was unsure if it was it or not. I was in the middle of doing work and my partner was the other side of London. I suddenly realised I needed to wash my hair so I had a bath, washed my hair, made a spag bol and put clean sheets on the bed! Then the cramps started and I rested.' Georgina Graham

'My waters started to leak at 4am, quickly followed by tightenings and an hour later I knew they were proper contractions! Hubby and I stared at each other in bed, like kids on Christmas morning – we were very excited!' Bev Samways

'I felt relief and excitement! And a pressure to keep the labour going. Wellies on, big hill climb, come home, sit down, contractions stop. Wellies back on, hill climb! I did it three times until it got dark then I resorted to hula hooping on the Wii Fit board, which was a good baby encouragement exercise!' Tessa Chapman

'My labour started when my waters broke at dawn, it woke me up. For an hour I shook from head to toe with adrenaline and anticipation, but the contractions didn't start for a while.' Amanda Twohey

'Exciting! It's happening! My body does know how to birth!' Katy Beale

3. The Niggling Phase

Midwives love this word: niggling. They use it to describe women in the very early part of labour, who are starting to feel those Braxton Hicks more strongly. We could also call this the 'Yes, Something IS *Finally* Flipping Happening Phase'. It really feels like everything could be getting going at last. Some women's waters break, but often this doesn't happen until much later in labour. But the tightenings in your bump will start to be harder to ignore, and you might think about timing the distance between them, either with an app or a good old-fashioned clock. If you are planning to give birth in a hospital or midwife-led unit (MLU), then you will normally be advised to wait until your tightenings or contractions are 30 to 60 seconds long and about 5 minutes apart before heading in. But don't be disappointed if this doesn't happen for a while – often the 'Niggling' phase can be very stop-start. Sleeping and eating are both great ideas in this phase, as you gather your energy for what is ahead.

What does it feel like?
Exciting, focusing, lower back pain, period pain, can still be very stop-start.

'I felt really agitated. What do I do? Sleep? Get in the pool? Do stuff to get ready? Eat?' Lora Willshaw

'All I wanted to do was lie on the sofa half asleep and use a contraction timing app – something I had repeatedly said I wouldn't do!' Cristina Freniche

'Both times I woke up in the early morning when it was still dark with gentle, cramping surges that I could no longer sleep through.' Nicola Snoad

'With my first baby I didn't really have any niggles at all, I just went straight into a rhythmical labour.' Claire Klymo

'There was an inordinate amount of going back and forth to the loo to poo! This was not what I expected, and I felt painful and crampy. I was sick too when things started to progress more. Gently swaying my hips helped.' Claire Kay

'I just felt so excited.' Fiona Jones

4. The Ramping Up Phase
Slowly but surely, the niggling phase gives way to something that feels a bit different, as labour gathers pace and 'ramps up'. You might find that the **tightenings**, surges or contractions demand your full attention, and that you begin to get into a rhythm or dance with them. For example, each time you feel one approach you might lean on the chest of drawers, rock back and forward, moan, and work your way through it until you feel it subside again. Then you might carry on with what you were doing. Remember, between surges you will feel completely normal and often, by this stage, very energised, happy, or

Pssst... a word about the 'Long Latent Phase'

Sometimes, the Niggling Phase can give way to the Ramping Up Phase and you can think, OK, here we go, but then ... it all stops. Then it can niggle and ramp up again ... and stop again. This experience, sometimes called a 'Long Latent Phase' or 'False Labour' (another negative label, cheers – um, if you feel like you are in labour, um, you are?!) can go on for a really long time, sometimes even days, and leave you feeling disheartened and exhausted before you've even really got going on the task of having a baby. Here are some tips if this happens to you:

1. **Trust in the process.** Know that this happens often to women and it is a perfectly common beginning to labour. Your body is getting ready in its own way – like an orchestra tuning up for the main performance!

2. **Try to stay rested and nourished.** Do what you can to keep calories on board and keep hydrated. Sleep or rest as much as possible. If lying down is uncomfortable, you may be able to snooze leaning on a pile of pillows or even a birth ball. If you cannot sleep, try comfort methods such as baths, hot water bottles, massage or hugs.

3. **Listen to your body.** You might be told to keep moving, go for walks, or bounce on your ball to get things going, but only do this if you feel like it. It's important to gather your strength, not wear yourself out.

4. **Get support.** Call in a loving team, for example family, or doula, to care for you and do everything for you (cooking, care of other children). Let others take over and just focus on yourself.

5. **Don't obsess over numbers.** Try not to pay too much attention to how many centimetres you may have dilated, or not, or how many hours or days you have been in this place of struggle. If you are examined, ask your midwife to tell you if she thinks baby is moving down, or if your cervix is thinning, as well as how dilated you are. Whatever her assessment, do not be disheartened: you will meet your baby soon.

6. **Remember oxytocin.** The hormone of labour and birth does not like counting contractions on mobile phone apps, but it does like cups of hot chocolate by candlelight. For more on this see page 128.

even a bit 'trippy' from the hormonal experience. If you're not giving birth at home you will probably travel during the Ramping Up Phase.

What does it feel like?
Exciting, dream-like, scary, intensifying, rhythmical, powerful, and like you are definitely going to have a baby!

'For me the contractions changed from period-type cramps to definite squeezes, and my belly got significantly harder than it had been doing before. I felt like I was all belly, and all my attention was there with these white hot sensations that began as tingles and rose to peaks of incredible power. I was just riding these fabulous waves of energy. It hurt, a lot, but I could handle it, I knew it was OK, it was pain with a purpose and I was a mama tiger!' Lyndsey Kindred

'I was trying to get the rhythm going, swaying, smiling and sinking into the labour cave inside my head.' Olga Danyluk-Singh

'On one side I felt more excited, on the other my mind was elsewhere, like in a dream.' Cristina Freniche

'I remembered I actually had to get a person out of me, and tried to concentrate on breathing.' Lora Willshaw

'This bit was interesting, it felt like, finally! Here is the labour I've been waiting to experience! I really enjoyed the shower and being by myself. I used breath from prenatal yoga, where the exhale is blown out of the mouth. This made it very manageable without getting tired.'
Jacquelyn Aurora, USA

'I loved this part for my second baby. I remember dancing and swaying in the kitchen to the radio, waiting for the midwife to arrive and just savouring each sensation.' Wendy Evans

5. The Cracking On Phase
Hold on to your hat, this is when it really gets interesting. You are totally, fully and unmistakably in the thickest, fullest and most intense part of labour. I've heard some midwives refer to this phase as 'Yahooing', and Miranda Hart's Chummy describes it as, 'when labour really gets its boots on'. Your contractions will probably come more

frequently, be more intense, and last longer. You will probably not feel like talking or doing anything else. You will be in the place that some people call 'Labour Land', utterly focused on riding the waves and staying afloat.

What does it feel like?

Later on in this chapter we'll talk about labour pain and how some people don't experience giving birth as painful. However, many people do find this part of labour really hard work and really intense. There is still some of the golden time between contractions, but they are closer together, and the peaks of them can be, well, cracking.

'I felt like I could see inside my body and see my baby moving down. I remember my husband trying to feed me melon and spitting it out behind the bed. I couldn't talk or acknowledge anybody, I was completely consumed.' Michelle Quashie

'I can remember a point where things changed, I began to roar through my contractions, a deep, guttural moaning vibration that was the only way to release the massive energy surging through me. I felt like I might take off, and the sounds I was making grounded me. I stayed on all fours, I swayed and rocked. After a while I needed a bit of relief and used the gas and just drifted between the rushes, spacey but focused too, flowing with my body. There was intense pain, but it was powerful energy I could lean into, work with and roar with.' Lyndsey Kindred

'I am a warrior. I am in control. I am power. This doesn't have power over me. One contraction more, one less until we meet our baby. Just taking it one at a time, battle after battle.' Olga Danyluk-Singh

'I felt a combination of pure panic, being in a different world, and being high as a kite from gas and air!' Cristina Freniche

'During my intense contractions I was focused fully on my breathing. In through my nose deeply, then out through my mouth noisily. When I did this my focus was entirely in my breath and I didn't feel the contractions as pain and could ride them. If I lost concentration I would suddenly find myself focused on the sharp overwhelming feelings in my cervix and it was too much. I had to pull myself back up to my head to regain control.' Verity Croft

'Everything external was forced out, an involuntary necessity – partner, light, noise, activity – I achieved this by squatting in a corner, facing it, with head lowered. Perfect!' Lisa Casson

'I had "back labour" the entire time. Making two fists and putting them behind my back against the wall, I moved in rhythm. I wanted my husband beside me, but wanted no touch at all. All consuming is how I would describe the feeling.' Vijaya Krishnan

'Primitive. I remember feeling like a strong primitive woman without inhibition. All care for others went out the window as I surrendered to the contractions, breathing instinctively and swaying in tune with my breaths. I loved birth.' Jules McKoy

'I could really distinctly feel my cervix opening – it was an amazing feeling! Contractions were very strong and definitely painful, but it was a manageable pain, completely unlike anything else... it felt productive. I felt a lot lower down in my womb. I could clearly tell when my cervix was fully open and my contractions changed to "pushing ones" – suddenly that pressure moved from lower down to the top of my womb and I could feel my muscles moving my baby down and out. Amazing!' Sarah Berryman

6. Transition

I've deliberately not talked about dilation until now because I really want to discourage you from worrying about measuring the opening of your cervix in centimetres and focus instead on the experience of being in labour. You may even wish to decline routine examinations to measure your dilation (see page 91). However, transition means you've reached full dilation, which is roughly around 10cm: the size of a bagel or a box of cheese triangles!

Transition is a time when everything changes, hence the very apt word – transition. You will feel this, and it will be happening in your hormones as oxytocin makes way for the adrenaline you need to wake you up from Labour Land and energise you enough to give birth. This shift from oxytocin to adrenaline may even cause you to feel 'fear' at this moment, but this doesn't mean that you cannot do it. It just means you *are* doing it.

What does it feel like?

This stage can feel hugely emotional: that you absolutely cannot go on, that you want a caesarean, that you cannot cope, or that you want to die. Transition is intense, but usually brief: it is like a wave of feelings that will wash over you and then pass away as all waves do.

'Transition for me during all three of my labours was the only time I doubted my body's ability. For a few minutes I completely panicked and considered pulling my knickers back on and running for the hills.'
Sophia Cannon

'I felt sweaty, shaky, shivery, and the overwhelming urge to be completely naked.' Sarah Shaw

'I felt terror. I actually let go of the gas and air to scream "I want to die".' Cristina Freniche

'As a midwife, I always called this "hammer time", as in "Will someone please hit me on the head with a hammer?". This is when women often start screaming for an epidural, or drugs, or ANYTHING that will separate them from this experience that has become seemingly "impossible to handle". I knew one day I would be on the receiving end as a birthing mother, and I certainly screamed for a hammer too! I reached out to my midwife, through my tears, and each one (I've had four births at home) shared the strength and wisdom necessary for me to trust my body and trust that I wasn't, in fact, going to die. The experience of consciously living through transition is an amazing source of pride and strength for women. It's a myth that we have to be physically "cut off" from the experience. We CAN do it.'
Elizabeth Soubelet

'All I could say was "Flipping Nora" over and over again. I don't know where that came from? Not one of my usual phrases.' Michelle Quashie

'I remember saying "I can't do it", even though throughout the whole pregnancy and labour I had been super positive. A few words from my partner, mum and the midwives helped me realise I definitely could.'
Chloe Eleanor Geake

'In transition I lost my mind for a moment. I felt an incredibly large contraction, and in a huge wave of intense pain I climbed the air trying

to escape my belly. I swore I couldn't do it, I begged them to make it stop, and when it was over, I could feel that my baby had dropped down a lot. It was really wild.' <u>Lyndsey Kindred</u>

7. The Rest and Be Thankful Phase

This doesn't happen for all women, but some experience this 'pause', dubbed the Rest and Be Thankful Phase by birth guru Sheila Kitzinger, but rather beautifully named the Quietude by midwife Whapio Diane Bartlett. For some women this phase lasts long enough to cause care providers concern that labour has 'stalled'. More often than not, it hasn't, and after these moments of gathering in fortitude and courage, the majority of women will make the leap of faith into the final phases of bringing a new human on to the earth.

What does it feel like?

A sudden, unexpected moment of calm, like somebody pressed the pause button on the rollercoaster.

'I had a rest and be thankful phase in my second birth. I quite clearly remember that I dropped my head down and drifted off for a few minutes. It felt like I went into myself and no one else in the room was there, I was kneeling in the pool. Then literally I woke and I knew what was to come and felt intense pressure.' <u>Tara Louise Luke</u>

'This was so lovely, a trance-like state.' <u>Lindsay Dalton</u>

'With our first little boy James everything literally just stopped... It was suggested that myself and my husband made the most of the rest. I was told "You're tired, your baby is tired, you just need to rest". We were both sent to bed. We had an hour of much needed "sleep" before it all kicked off again.' <u>Emma-Jane Cunningham</u>

'There were no rest phases for me in either of my births.' <u>Klaire Clymo</u>

'I had a rest and be thankful stage with my first baby. I had no idea what it was until after the birth. All I knew was that I absolutely HAD to lie down, and nothing was going to stop me. I had a very bossy midwife who wanted me up, but I was having none of it and wanted to drop off to sleep. I lay down for about 20 minutes until they dragged me up. I wish I'd had a more relaxed midwife who knew this was a rest and be

thankful stage, and just let me go with it.' Rebecca Lush

'Oh good, relief suddenly. A chance to go to the toilet... I needed a lot of support to get to the bathroom. But a short-lived feeling as I then realised it's the baby coming now!" Christina Pelentrides

'It was a moment of calm and clarity. I put my contact lenses in for the post-birth photos at this point!' Susan Last

8. The Pushing Phase

Some people can take up to two hours, sometimes longer, to push their baby out, while others, particularly those who experience the Foetus Ejection Reflex (see page 98), might go from fully dilated to baby in arms in a matter of minutes. Some women like guidance and direction at this point, whereas others prefer to spiral inwards again and listen to their body. Some find that they don't actually have to 'push' at all, and that the effort is all completely involuntary, like sneezing. You will still have contractions in the Pushing Phase, but they will feel different because you will feel compelled to push while they are happening, and some women prefer this more active phase of their labour. Like all of the phases, the Pushing Phase is often blended in to the other neighbouring phases, so what you might find is that, during the Cracking On Phase, you suddenly start to feel a bit different during contractions, or make different noises. A midwife might ask you, "Are you feeling a bit 'pushy'?", and if you are, you will instantly know what she means. This 'pushy' feeling will build and become more intense, usually so that you cannot resist it.

What does it feel like?

This active phase of labour can make you feel like being intensely quiet or roaring like a lioness. The physical sensations as your baby descends, through the cervix and down your vagina, are some of the most extremely intense bodily experiences you will ever have. Some can feel themselves stretching and widening. Some feel their baby rotate and move, moment by moment. Love it or hate it, you will certainly never forget this part of labour.

'I LOVED pushing! I delivered my 9lbs 13.5oz baby boy standing over the edge of my bed. With every surge I lifted my head and threw every ounce of my being into bringing him down and out to me. I remember

my boyfriend's eyes were the only thing I could look at and he stared right back like we were the only two souls in the world. I'll never forget how frighteningly powerful, beautiful and determined I felt in those moments, it still makes me so emotional and proud.' Jen Muir

'It felt overwhelming and way out of my control.' Sarah Caldwell

'I love this stage, it's been my favourite with both of my children, so primal! Just shutting out everything but my body's signals. I was in the birthing pool by then, and just let my body twist and move exactly as it wanted to, let the bearing down happen almost by itself, I was so far away that when she was crowning I had to shout 'It's coming, it's coming!', as I wasn't sure if anyone else realised (they totally did, I was just unaware in labour land!) Then they encouraged me to slow down and just let her come slowly and her head did, then whoosh, her whole body just slid out super fast, the most bizarre feeling in the world!' Lyndsey Kindred

'For my first it took about two hours. I pushed and pushed and pushed and he kept bouncing back up inside of me, I felt desperate to get this finished, I was slightly worried I was doing something wrong and I was exhausted. I absolutely could only push, my body was doing it and I couldn't help but push with it, I was very worried I was going to birth out of my bottom! My second baby, I felt liberated and powerful, letting my body do what it needed to do, but as with each of my labours, pushing was the most painful /intense part. My third birth, once again, my body completely took over with an intense poo-like pushing and he was coming fast. I had no fear this time, but was overwhelmed by intensity and zinging with nervous excitement.' Wendy Evans

'It was like my body was heaving like it would when you are about to be sick but in the opposite direction. I couldn't stop it. My belly was convulsing, the midwife was telling me I'm not ready to push but I couldn't stop it. Less than 10 minutes later I was holding my son.' Michelle Quashie

'To start it felt like I needed to poo a cannon ball! Then pushing was something that happened to me, rather than me having any control over it; I could not have prevented it, nor aided it! My body literally took charge, even down to what position I was in (on all fours, bum in the air, head and arms on floor!). It felt primal and yet I KNEW everything was totally fine. In fact the pain of expulsion contractions was much more

manageable than dilation contractions. My senses were heightened and yet at the same time I couldn't interact with the outside world at all. In a way it was like the ultimate meditative or mindfulness experience: existing purely in the moment on a completely physical level. Amazing!'
Eleanor Hayes

'Your body just takes over. You can feel your body pushing your baby out and you don't have to do anything other than surrender to the moment. It's just gorgeous.' Suzy Ashworth

'The hardest work I've ever done.' Nyomi Winter

9. Crowning

Many women fear this part of giving birth, sometimes affectionately named the Ring of Fire. For many, there is a very strong burning sensation as the widest part of the baby's head sits momentarily in the opening of your vagina. You are stretched wide, and some women will tear or graze at this point (see page 229). But not all women report stinging or burning while their baby is crowning. It's different for everyone, and the good news is that if you are one of the women who does not enjoy crowning, it is usually over very quickly.

What does it feel like?
Really being stretched very wide, and for some a burning or stinging sensation.

'It was surprising, I felt scared and then amazed it was happening.'
Lindsay Dalton

'The only way to describe it is it feels like pooing a melon and you are going to rip in half! But you know there is no going back and you just want it done.' Claire Elliott

'I put my hand down and felt my baby's head emerging – one of the most amazing things ever! Completely instinctively, I gently touched her head from that moment until she slipped out a minute later into my arms.'
Sarah Berryman

'I can remember that bit quite vividly, suddenly realising she was almost here and almost wanting it to slow down, but my body just powering her

out. It's exquisite pain, I just had to go towards it, into it and through it, even when spikes of fear that "this was really it" kicked in. I managed to slow her for the last bit, but she really wanted to be born! I felt incredibly powerful bringing her down.' Lyndsey Kindred

'The burning sensation: like when you have a urinary tract infection, it burns like that, it reaches a threshold and then it's amazing because your body is so sensitive there you actually get to feel every detail of your baby's face before even seeing it! It literally is imprinting in your brain a tactile image!' Nahomie Hann

'At the crowning juncture I felt the vaginal opening stretching to its widest point. My first instinct was to hold back! But luckily my mind recognised that this was a point to be carefully navigated. At the next push, I focused my energy on slowly but steadily pushing through that burning feeling while trying to stay relaxed. I was afraid, but I knew fighting against these sensations was not going to take me where I wanted to go. A little bit of surrender goes a long way, and the next thing I knew, my son was out and I was holding him.' Maureen Whitman

'It was like eating chillies with cracked lips.' Shelley Dawn

10. The Head Being Born

As your baby crowns, one or two more pushes – which your midwife may or may not guide you through – will bring their head into the world.

What does it feel like?

One final stretching sensation, and then often a huge sense of relief, as you know the hardest part of labour is behind you.

'Like the biggest poo ever.' Leanne O'Donnell

'This was the only moment of panic I had – when I looked down and saw a head between my legs. I don't remember feeling pain. The panic was because I could see my baby – she was nearly fully out – and I hoped she was OK!' Katy Beale

'Streeeeeeeetch, ahhhhhhhhh, awkward relief... but sat there with the biggest, warmest baby head between your legs... whoa! Then the longest wait in the world for the next contraction.' Wendy Evans

'I remember thinking "Thank God, the baby is nearly here!" I was so excited. I knew within minutes my baby would be in my arms. A very special moment.' Chloe Eleanor Geake

'Incredible, and it is so strange when you have a few minutes' gap until the next contraction, with a head hanging out of you! My husband can really clearly remember seeing our first daughter's head turning as her shoulders started to emerge, in that classic twist babies do.' Rebecca Lush

11. The Body Being Born

There is usually a pause after the head has been born, while you wait for the next surge to give birth to the body. After the hard work of the head, the body feels like a slippery eel, moving out of you with one final sensation of release.

What does it feel like?

Sometimes you will feel your baby wriggle to move out of you with the final contraction. Giving birth to their body is hugely triumphant and relieving. It can feel very sensual, a fantastic physical experience, perhaps even orgasmic.

'This was an amazing slithery feeling, like when you have a really thick gloopy sauce in a pot and you turn it upside down and it suddenly just flops into the saucepan?! Pure relief!' Jules Bambridge

'I felt his shoulders, elbows and body come out – it was bizarre.' Georgina Graham

'Oh my, that amazing feeling of schlooooping as the whole body slides out and you suddenly feel empty, it's an indescribable sensation!' Verity Croft

'Like cooked pasta... They just slippy slid out on a wave of relief and sheer joy!' Jen Muir

'I will never forget the feeling of the limbs leaving my body. It's still so clear 15 years on. The shoulders, the arms, the legs, even the feet. I felt immediately empty and that he wasn't solely "mine" any more, he could be seen and held by all. My "bump" was now a fully exposed human. I felt initially redundant and a bit sad I now had to share him!' Claire Elliott

'Oh wowzas! Total and utter release but with a little bit of "is that it?!" especially after the intensity leading up to that moment. With my first I genuinely said "is that a baby!?"' Nicola Snoad

'It was a big, strange, slithery sensation (actually totally painless – but weird!) And there was my baby, born right into my hands. Incredible, I've never felt anything like it.' Samantha Norman

12. Baby in Arms

Yes, you've done it! Your baby has been born! At the moment of birth you might reach down to take your baby and bring baby up to you. Other times a midwife might pass you your baby. Some prefer to leave their baby for a moment and take a look at them before picking them up. Some leave their baby on their stomach and let them find their own way to the breast in a move known as the Breast Crawl. Now is the time for vital skin-to-skin (see page 109), and remember, there is no rush to cut the cord! (See page 103.)

What does it feel like?

It's a moment of triumph for many, this magical moment of meeting your son or daughter for the first time. For others, the magic comes later on and they need some time to take stock. Physically, some feel hugely energised and on top of the world, while others feel utterly spent. Once the euphoria of meeting their baby has passed, many women describe feeling a little 'unfinished', as the body knows it still has work to do expelling the placenta.

'I felt bliss and love but then shock and an uncontrollable shaking set in.' Eva Bay

'Pure relief, gratitude and happiness, but also total exhaustion. I felt overwhelmed as so much had just happened and was happening. So much to take in.' Nyomi Winter

'I felt a massive sense of achievement; the waiting had come to an end and my baby was here with me! We didn't even check the sex of the baby for a good few minutes. It was a beautiful moment.' Chloe Eleanor Geake

'Absolute and complete shock and numb. But that first look where they lock eyes onto you? Priceless. One hundred per cent Disney moment

with birds flying and deer peering through the window!' Claire Elliott

'I remember asking "Have I done it?" and then slowly realising that I had! I kept repeating "I've done it, I've done it!" as I kissed my husband and midwives repeatedly. It took me a few moments to realise that my baby was still between my legs as I knelt on the bed. I reached down, claimed him as mine, and triumphantly lifted him to my breast.' Joy Horner

'Exhausted – what, I have to look after a baby now?' Alex Heath

'Always the surprise that I actually have a baby in my arms! Up until that point it's so hard to believe that by the end of these 9 months there comes a human. On holding both my girls for the first time I let out a primal sort of howling sob, never made it before or since!' Nicola Snoad

'She was born into my hands and I lifted her to my chest. I blurted out "Oh my God, you are the most beautiful thing I've ever seen!" She was a kind of lilac colour at first, her eyes were open and she was looking right at my face. At that moment I never wanted to let her go.' Samantha Norman

13. The Placenta Coming Out

Just when you thought you'd utterly nailed it, you realise you've still got one more job left to do, pushing out your placenta. The good news is that after a baby this feels like a teeny tiny friendly little portion of jelly. Your midwives will talk you through it, and once you're done, you really are done this time, and you can sink back on your pillows with your baby snugged in tight feeling like an absolute goddess.

What does it feel like?

Usually easy peasy. Sometimes quite enjoyable. And frankly, a bit weird.

'Like pulling out a tampon. A real "aahhh that's better" moment! I was in awe of the size and appearance of it.' Nicola Snoad

'All my placentas felt to me like another baby coming out... size wise, they felt very big and I had to give them a good push out. With the first one I was badgered to take the injection after waiting an hour, but for the next two I delivered them by myself, standing over my loo at home. The last one I delivered all on my own and checked it over myself, it felt

good and right to be able to have that moment to myself and be curious on my own. I loved looking at my placenta!' Wendy Evans

'It took so much longer than I expected both times. With baby number two it took an hour; longer than the whole of my very fast labour! I found it frustrating and exhausting to continue having contractions. I wish I had realised how much longer it could take when you're already tired and fed up of pushing!!' Shelly Dawn

'With both my girls I don't even remember the placenta arriving, I was too involved with staring at the baby in my arms in complete wonder.' Saira Tubb

'It took a while for them to get it out and I INSISTED on seeing it and was surprised by how huge it was. My husband looked like he was going to pass out as it was delivered. He told me two years later he had no idea anything else was supposed to come out and he thought they'd pulled a lung or my liver out. I still crack up laughing when I think about how uninformed he was and how scared he must have been.' Wendy Evans

'It felt like nothing compared to the baby, and very small!' Georgina Graham

14. The Tea and Toast Phase

All being well, you are holding your baby, skin-to-skin. There may be a midwife or two taking an occasional peek at your nether regions, but frankly, you don't really give a damn. If you do need stitches you will get them now, but, proving for every yin there's a yang, you'll also get the best cup of tea and slice of hot buttered toast you've ever had in your life. After that you can move straight to the champers. Even if it is 7.45am. Hey, it's five o'clock somewhere.

What does it feel like?
Champion.

'I remember grinning. Just like that. With all my three babies I didn't cry, I was just purely happy and grateful I got the birth I wished for, baby is here and we get to breastfeed. A new chapter began.' Olga Danyluk-Singh

'When my baby was put on my chest I was like awww he's so slippery and slimy but I bloody love him. I remember everything else apart from him almost being out of focus, like we were in a weird little bubble. It's not very often that my mind is still but at that moment all I was thinking about was this slimy little creature that I'd been dying to meet for sooooo long and he was finally here!' Leah Freeman

'We had waited five years and three miscarriages for our baby. I didn't realise it until afterwards, but I actually doubted all the way through labour that I was going to have a baby. I subconsciously read into things my team was doing and saw danger when there was none, but managed to keep calm and trust them. There was this moment, after he was born, where I looked at him and realised this was indeed my baby, the one we'd been waiting for. Thanks to my doula, I have a picture of this exact moment. It shows me overwhelmed with emotion. I remember the grief and the heartache pouring out while the love poured in.' Michelle Gossen

'I felt huge surges of joy, pride, relief, disbelief – I couldn't have imagined how it felt being handed my new babe – but it was just so exactly right that he fitted in my tired shaking arms and I soaked him in physically and emotionally, every bit of his perfect body, his gentle calm reaction to being with us. It was like we'd just had a mysterious magic box opened in front of us and light filled the room. Everything was still and my surroundings faded and all I could see was him. I could not stop smelling his head – this went on for days – I felt like a cat, it was like a drug, I couldn't get enough!' Tortie Rye

'With my first, I felt traumatised, exposed, exhausted, weak, shocked and grateful it was over and my boy was OK. With my second, I felt like a goddess, loved and in love, safe in our home, physically drained and sore but triumphant.' Lyndsey Kindred

'That first hour was just magic, complete magic. I was sky high on endorphins and felt like I was wonder woman and could do anything!' Emma Mills

'Perfection. You just lie there marvelling at your baby and how bloody amazing it is that you've done it.' Suzy Ashworth

'Our amazing midwife didn't interfere in our time with our baby at all after his birth. Those hours my partner and I spent skin-to-

skin, smelling him, nursing, kissing him and each other are the most dreamlike I've ever experienced. Even my two elder sons were able to hold and fall in love with their little brother before he was weighed and checked. We will never forget that time.' Jen Muir

What does caesarean birth feel like?

The 'in-labour caesarean'

If you give birth by caesarean, you might still experience some or almost all of the fourteen stages of labour! Sometimes the decision to give birth surgically is made very late on in your labour, and you may have got all the way to being fully dilated. Birth pioneer Michel Odent suggests that this might be positive, because, if the birth is not induced, we can be sure that the baby is ready to be born. He also suggests that the experience of labour might be good for the mother and the baby in ways that we don't yet understand, as well as in ways that we do – for instance, we know that hormones play an important part in bonding, and that being in labour is a unique hormonal experience. Evidence also shows that your chances of a vaginal birth if you go on to have another baby (VBAC, see page 236), are higher if you have experienced labour before your caesarean. For these reasons, some women choose to wait for their labour to begin naturally, even if they are planning a caesarean. Once labour has begun, they then attend hospital for the birth in theatre.

The 'non-labour caesarean'

You may not wish to have an 'in-labour caesarean' and the day and time of the birth might be completely planned in advance, or you may find yourself suddenly being told you need a caesarean due to concerns about your health or the health of your baby. In these cases you won't experience many of the stages of labour, although, even with the best-laid plans, you may have a few niggles before the day, and you will almost certainly get to experience most women's favourite birth moment, when your baby is placed in your arms.

Whether you have an 'in-labour caesarean' or a 'non-labour caesarean', you are likely to feel quite anxious or scared before or during the birth. There are lots of ways that you can help yourself to feel more calm, in control and at the centre of the experience, for example by using breathing or visualisation techniques (see page 138), or by requesting a woman-centred caesarean (see page 208). It's also really important not to forget your wishes for caesarean birth when you make your birth plan (see page 116).

'Walking to theatre was very odd knowing that I was walking towards a huge operation that also happened to be the birth of my baby. I think that gets forgotten.' Kim Kidney

'The spinal was uncomfortable but not for long. The feeling of the numbness spreading up your body is like slipping into a lovely hot tub. There was no feeling for the incision, and the actual delivery felt like someone was washing dishes inside my tummy.' Crystal Steinberg

Vivienne Cruddace, from Scotland, describes her caesarean birth

Waiting for the cold epidural to trickle down my back into my legs, in a chilly theatre, the warmth of a hand on mine is welcome. I'm calm but terrified, excited but scared of letting go, anxious of handing my body over to these people to open and deliver my baby from. The senior midwife holds my hand until we are ready to begin, telling me what I will and won't feel, but I'm not really listening. The drapes are down, and the incision is made. While they are telling me what they are doing and what is coming next, I feel nothing but impatient anticipation for them to bring my baby out. Quickly, there are arms round my shoulders and I am gently lifted a little to be greeted by the sight of my daughter appearing into the world. The cold, blue theatre is filled with golden light and sound as she lets us know she is here, and her hot, vernix-covered body is placed against my chest. The rest of the world slips away, and it's just us two, breathing each other in, heart-to-heart, skin-to-skin, fluid between one person and two. The rest of my body is of no concern to me now, and I am blissfully unaware as they close and prepare to take me to recovery. And then it's all over – in the space of an hour I have gone from walking around, finishing my online Sainsbury's shop, to having a baby, our daughter, in my arms.

'Once I had had my spinal anaesthetic my blood pressure dropped a bit making me feel cold and I began to shake uncontrollably. The theatre staff were gorgeous and brought me an extra blanket for my shoulders.'
Nicola Nelson

'My surgeon was happy to have the drape as low as possible and talked me through the whole birth. I'd heard of a caesarean feeling like someone is doing the washing up on the other side of the drape, but I barely remember myself being moved around at all. I often think that this was due to having the drape lowered. I wasn't disconnected from any movement I suppose; it wasn't an abstract experience.' Nicola Nelson

'They have to put a lot of pressure on the top of your uterus – I wasn't expecting this! Someone was leaning on me and although it wasn't painful I did feel a bit squashed.' Caroline Smith

'Once he was out they took him for a few moments and then popped him skin-to-skin (I'd requested this in my 'just in case' birth plan) and he stayed there for a while. I wasn't that aware of the surgery at this point as I was so infatuated.' Julie Thompson

Florence Wilcock, consultant obstetrician at Kingston Hospital NHS Foundation Trust, talks us through some of the details of caesarean birth

The majority of caesarean sections in the UK will be done under a spinal anaesthetic – that is, numb from the nipples downwards. It's a peculiar feeling as you can feel touch, but not pain. It means that women will be conscious and aware of people milling around them, which can be daunting, but it also means they are awake and ready to meet their new baby.
We tilt women lying on the operating table slightly to their left to keep the bump of the baby off the major blood vessels; this prevents dizziness from low blood pressure. In the maternity theatres at my Trust you look up at butterflies and cherry blossom on the ceiling; something nice to focus on while you wait for your baby to arrive. I know this is unusual and we are lucky, but there is nothing to stop you tucking your favourite picture or photo into your birthing bag so that you have something familiar and relaxing to look at.

Who's who?

It might seem odd that at the start of the operation, everyone in the theatre will introduce themselves to one another. It isn't that we have never met, but it's part of the World Health Organisation (WHO) safe surgery checklist. So, who are all these people around you, what are their roles, and why are there so many of them?

Anaesthetist: At least one, sometimes two; these are doctors who will administer the anaesthetic and monitor you closely during the surgery. They will be standing just by your head and often chat to you and reassure you as the operation progresses.

Operating Department Practitioner (ODP): at least one; their role is to assist the anaesthetist, getting and checking the required drugs, drips or equipment. The anaesthetist cannot work without one being present.

Obstetricians: at least two; one will be performing the caesarean section (the surgeon) the other will be assisting (the assistant), for example cutting stitches, holding instruments.

Midwife: At least one; to support the woman and help her with her newborn baby when it arrives.

Scrub nurse or midwife: At least one; to check and count all needles, stitches and instruments and to hand them to the surgeon when needed.

Midwifery assistant or runner: to double check the swab and instrument count with the scrub midwife or nurse, and 'run' to get any additional equipment required. They are not 'scrubbed up' so can go in and out of theatre to fetch things.

Paediatrician: asked to attend any 'emergency' situation or if there are known concerns about the baby.

So in theatre there is a minimum of seven people caring for any woman, all with specific tasks to perform. Any complication may result in us calling in extra members of the team.

The woman will be on the operating table with her birth partner by her side and the anaesthetist and ODP close at hand. She can often choose the music she would like her baby to be born to. The anaesthetist needs to monitor her heart with sticky labels, but these can be put on her back and her gown left loose, leaving her chest free and ready for skin-to-skin with her baby. A sterile drape will be placed over her bump and this is usually used to make a 'screen' so that she doesn't see any surgery; however, we usually drop this when the baby is ready to be born.

Many hospitals are starting to explore optimal cord clamping (waiting to clamp the cord) and passing the baby straight to the mother if the baby is in good condition. Both are possible, if care is taken not to contaminate the sterile surgical area and the surgeon is confident no harm, such as excessive bleeding from the womb, is occurring. Surgical lights need to be on so the surgeon can see clearly and operate safely, but I know one anaesthetist who works in a hospital where the rest of the theatre lights can be dimmed. The mum and new baby can be enjoying skin-to-skin while the rest of the operation proceeds. Weighing and checking babies can be done at this time, but also can be done later on.

Traditionally, if we operate on a woman under general anaesthetic (asleep), her birth partner has not been in theatre. Recently on several occasions I have challenged this, so that the baby is welcomed to the world with at least one of its family present and awake, rather than by a group of strangers caring for the unconscious mother. There are safety considerations, but it is possible. However kind and caring staff are, they are no replacement for a birth partner whom the mother has chosen to support her in the intimacy of birth.

I hope I have given you a brief glimpse of life in a maternity theatre. As an obstetrician I am privileged to help bring many women and babies together for those special first moments. The emotions are always different for me –sometimes the parents are a couple I know very well and have bonded with over months or years; sometimes a woman I have only just met has had to put her absolute trust in me immediately. The theatre atmosphere can range from almost party-like jollity to quiet intimacy. Every birth is different, and every birth is extremely special, just like births that happen in a less clinical environment. Each birth will stay with that woman forever.

How much does giving birth actually hurt?

Ever heard horror stories about birth lasting hours and hours, and formed a mental picture of a sweaty woman writhing in non-stop-agony, like something mediaeval was occurring? Yeah, I bet you have. But hold on, let's look at things from a fresh angle, and do some maths.

The average first stage of labour lasts about eight hours. I'm going to talk averages here for the purpose of our mental arithmetic, and of course, just as people can vary, so can these numbers. Bear with me, this is going somewhere – honest.

So. It's an eight-hour first stage. That's the bit when your cervix is dilating.

For the first hour, you might have a contraction every 20 minutes. That's the bit that hurts.

These contractions might last on average 60 seconds.

So that's three in the first hour, lasting a minute each. That's three minutes of contractions.

In hour two, they might come every 10 minutes. So that's six contractions in the second hour of labour.

By hour three, they might be coming '2 in 10', that's two every 10 minutes. So that's 12 contractions in hour three.

For the next five hours of labour, things might really ramp up, so you are having '3 in 10'. That gives you a total of 18 an hour, which in five hours adds up to 90 contractions.

So. In your eight-hour first stage, that's a total of 111 minutes of contractions. That's only 23 per cent of your time spent having contractions. The rest of the time, the other 369 minutes, the other 77 per cent, is entirely pain free!

And the news gets better.

Not every second of the 60-second contraction is horribly painful. Most women only find the 'peak' of the contraction really tough, and that lasts about 20 seconds. Of your eight-hour first stage, only 37 minutes will be spent at the peak of contractions. That's just 7.7 per cent.

So. That's 7.7 per cent of labour time that really, really hurts. 15.3 per cent moving towards or away from the peak of the contraction. And 77 per cent of labour that is pain free.

What a headline that would make! And yet nobody ever seems to talk about birth in these terms. Nobody tells you about the time between contractions, which makes up the vast majority of labour, during which you will feel completely awesome. The huge rush of hormones around your body, and the general excitement of the occasion, means that you will quite literally be glowing with vitality and positive energy. Yet nobody ever tells you this.

How does this affect us, as women, as we approach labour, and in labour itself? With all this talk of pineapples out of nostrils and soap opera images of women in distress, is it any wonder that many of us are full of dread and can only think about which pain relief option we are going to go for? Pain in labour can easily become our sole focus, and of course our expectations shape our reality.

If someone raises a stick in the air and utters the phrase 'This is going to really hurt' – what do we do? We tense our body in anticipation of the worst. We put all of our focus on the part of the body that's about to be hit. And we feel afraid, and distressed. A doctor in the 1950s called Grantly Dick-Read called this the 'Fear-Tension-Pain' cycle. It's a bit of a no-brainer really.

Anaesthetists administering epidurals report that sometimes, if a woman thinks the drugs have been given, even if they haven't yet, she will have a better experience with the next contraction, sometimes reporting it to be entirely pain-free. We cannot over-estimate the power of the mind in labour.

And there are women, of course, who report 'pain free' labours. When you talk to these rare nymphs, it's interesting to note the language they use. Words like 'intense', and 'powerful' recur again and again, suggesting that it is perhaps the way that these women are thinking about the sensations of labour that is different, rather than the sensations themselves.

Some women ban any talk of pain from their birth room, referring to contractions as 'surges' or 'rushes' and asking that they are not offered pain relief, but are given it if they request it. For obvious reasons, they don't even like the term 'pain relief', preferring to talk about 'coping strategies' or 'comfort measures'. And they don't want to hear someone say, 'Would you like an epidural?', because this might have the subtext of, 'You don't look like you're coping very well', and undermine their confidence. The importance of words is also emphasised by childbirth expert Penny Simkin, who stresses the vital distinction between 'pain' and 'suffering'. The former is an unpleasant physical sensation, while the latter is more about being overwhelmed, out of control and helpless.

'Many women "suffer" in childbirth', Simkin writes, 'And it's because they're not respected, or kindly treated, they don't have the tools to cope, or they feel unloved, or alone. If a woman crosses the line from "pain" into "suffering" in childbirth, we've failed her.' Or as another birth expert, American midwife Ina May Gaskin, would put it: 'If a woman doesn't look like a goddess in labour, someone isn't treating her right.'

How you will experience labour and how much it will 'hurt' is not a question I can answer, but what I can tell you is that it is hugely different from woman to woman, and from labour to labour, and that the best thing you can do is just to prepare your mind and body as best you can, and then 'suck it and see'. Your labour may be longer than my eight-hour example, or your baby might be in a difficult position. You might have great support for the first few hours, but then a change of shift might mean you feel a bit lost and start to struggle. If you feel you cannot cope, opt for pain relief and don't beat yourself up about it. Birth is not a competition.

I do, however, suggest that you open your mind up to the idea that labour and birth is about much more than pain, and that the current focus on how agonising it is, probably isn't doing us any favours. And even if the peak of contractions is absolute mind-bending torture, remember: this only takes up on average 7.7 per cent of your labour.

Because labour is 77 per cent pain free! You heard it here first.

What about the nightmare labour from hell? Do the maths for that, clever clogs!

OK, let's imagine there's no fluffy-wuffy time – lighting candles, face-timing your bestie, or making cookies. You draw the short straw, and get one of those labours (extremely rare, but nevertheless possible) where you go straight off the blocks at top speed and have four contractions every 10 minutes from start to finish, and the whole thing lasts 36 hours. I bet that wouldn't be 77 per cent pain free, I hear you cry.

Actually, the maths is still surprisingly positive.

If you're having a one-minute contraction, four times every 10 minutes, for 36 hours, that's 864 minutes spent in pain, out of 2,160 minutes of labour. 40 per cent contractions. 60 per cent pain free.

The extra tough peak of contractions will take up only around 13 per cent of your labour. Heading up to the peak and back down again will take up 27 per cent of your time. The other 60 per cent of your time – you are not in pain.

Of course, that's not to say that this kind of labour wouldn't be knackering, and there are also some labours where the pain is completely relentless. If your baby is in a tricky position, for example 'back to back', or you are feeling very scared or unsupported, you may find that there is no break from the pain. It's important to note, though, that in a straightforward labour, relentless agony is not normal. In these instances, knowing more about Optimal Foetal Positioning can help (see page 133), and, if it's unbearable, opioids or epidural can give you the break that you are craving.

Chapter 3

An A to Z of 'coping strategies' and 'comfort measures' for labour
(or, if you prefer, 'pain relief')

Active Birth

Staying active in your labour is one great way to feel more comfortable. Find the positions that feel right for you (see page 135), and work them, girlfriend. Often women find they develop a ritual of movement to deal with contractions, moving into a certain position each time they feel them approaching; rocking, vocalising, and then resting when they subside. Janet Balaskas, who created the idea of 'active birth' in the 1980s, felt that it applied to more than just physical positions – it was also a state of mind, and the choice to be 'active' rather than 'passive' in the birth experience.

Bottle – Hot Water

Heat applied to the lower back can be soothing and comforting. Try a hot water bottle with a nice soft cover, or a lavender wheat bag. Others prefer ice packs or bags of frozen peas. Another technique used by some midwives and doulas involves applying *very* hot flannels to the lower back during contractions: could this be the origin of the age-old call for 'Hot water and towels!'? Use with caution, as you obviously don't want to start motherhood with first-degree burns.

Clary Sage

Known as 'nature's gas and air', some women swear that a good sniff of this essential oil on a tissue during labour can make you feel beautifully floaty. Be aware that it's not advised to use clary sage before you reach full term, as it is said to be powerful enough to induce labour. Other essential oils that work well in labour are lavender, jasmine and citrus scents like mandarin and lemon. Use in an oil burner, on a hanky, or added to plain massage oil such as olive or almond. Don't add to the birth pool water, as if you hate it you'll be stuck with it.

Doula/Support

Don't underestimate the pain-relieving effects of feeling that someone is 100 per cent 'with' you in labour. A Cochrane review that pooled the results of 22 trials involving over 15,000 women found that simply having continuous support from the same person in labour leads to less need for pain relief (and fewer interventions, and better outcomes for mums and babies). And amazingly, this continuous support was found to be most effective if that support person was neither a member of hospital staff, nor from the woman's social network – in other words, a doula (see page 153).

Epidural

Most people have heard of this option, and it's become so strongly associated with birth that many women (and a fair few men!) hold the view that birth is not desirable, or even possible, without it. Essentially, it's a local anaesthetic that is administered by an anaesthetist using a needle, which is inserted in between the bones of your lower spine. A thin plastic tube called a catheter is then fed through the hollow needle and the tube is taped to your back, allowing the dose of the drug to be topped up as necessary. You can have a 'mobile' or 'low dose' epidural, in which anaesthetic is mixed with opioids allowing you more mobility, or a 'full epidural', which is a total block.

Advantages: if you are really not coping, it will usually completely stop the pain. With a mobile epidural you should still be able to move and have some sensation of your baby being born.

Disadvantages: you're more likely to have an instrumental delivery. You may need a catheter to help you urinate. You may have reduced sensations of your baby being born and will often, but not always, end up on your back on a bed being told what to do.

Flick The Bean

Masturbation in labour is a bit of a taboo subject, but many women report that it is a great way to either get labour going or to take them to a great, sensual place during surges or contractions. It can take a bit of a mental leap to think about labour in such positive, sexual terms. But not only will clitoral or nipple stimulation in labour get the oxytocin flowing, it might actually... feel nice?! What's to lose?

Gas And Air

Entonox, or 'gas and air', is a mixture of nitrous oxide (laughing gas) and oxygen. You will be offered it to inhale through a mouthpiece and you can have it at home or in the hospital or birth centre. You can use it during water birth too. Because it's inhaled it enters the body quickly, and also leaves quickly, so if you don't like the feeling it gives you, you won't be stuck with it for long. Some women swear by it and, once parenting gets into full swing, get a little canister installed in their kitchen so that they can have a quick drag at kids' suppertime or when they can't find the shoes for the school run. Others dislike it intensely and say it makes them dry-mouthed, nauseous or woozy.

Hypnobirthing

Many women find it helpful to prepare for labour using this technique, which involves deep relaxation, visualisation and an appreciation of the mind-body connection. Women who use birth hypnosis often report finding labour very manageable, or even pain-free, although there are no guarantees. If you're interested you can take classes or just purchase a CD or MP3. For more info see page 144.

Inhale, Exhale, Repeat

Breathing in labour has become a bit of a cliché since the 1970s, when women leant on their beardy and slightly awkward husbands in antenatal classes and puffed and sighed their way through imaginary contractions. But breathing calmly and deeply is a great way of centring yourself and gaining a sense of confidence and control – whether you are in labour or in the waiting room for a job interview. Practice in pregnancy: a yoga or meditation class is a good place to start, or just try deep relaxing breaths – in through the nose, out through the mouth – as you fall asleep each night.

Joke Around

A sense of humour in labour is highly recommended. It's a bit like going camping. If you think you are going to get through the experience while retaining your usual poise and Kardashian contouring, then you need a reality check. Like camping, giving birth involves getting down and dirty, letting go of many of the trappings of western 21st-century life, and some mild to moderate discomfort. And I'm sorry to say there's no compensatory barbequed sausages or wine in a plastic mug either. Laughing may therefore be essential for survival. It can also relieve pain by releasing beta endorphins (the brain's natural 'morphine'), perhaps why it's known as 'the best medicine'.

Kissing

Making out with your partner can be a great way to get labour going, and some women report that deep and passionate kissing can be just the thing during the intensity of contractions. Some say that 'the same energy that got the baby in, can get the baby out'. Others will tell you that the relaxed open mouth of a kiss will help your cervix to dilate effectively. Nothing to lose and everything to gain by trying this one.

Low Lights, Low Noise

Keeping the room dimly lit and quiet will allow you to focus and let your mammalian hormones flow. This gives you the best chance of staying on top of contractions. Interruptions, bright lights, sudden noise or irritating chitchat can all make it more difficult to cope with the intensity of labour.

Massage

Your partner, doula or midwife can massage you in labour, although you are unlikely to be interested in a gentle neck rub – what most labouring women seem to want is hard counter-pressure applied to their lower back during contractions. Essential oils can be part of the mix, and some doulas and midwives will use acupressure points to relieve pain or encourage labour to get moving. Some will use a 'hip press' – this involves squeezing your hip bones while you are standing or on all fours, to relieve pain and help open up the pelvis. Another technique is known as 'shaking the apple tree' and involves vigorously massaging the buttocks and upper thighs as if you were trying to make a ripe apple fall! Again, this is both to relieve pain and encourage progress. You might like to encourage your birth partner to research and practise some of these techniques – there is plenty of information and short films online. (Search for 'labour hip press' and 'labour shaking the apples'.)

Nourishment

Have a selection of food and drinks as part of your birth bag (see page 174) and keep up your intake of calories and fluid during labour. Low blood sugar or dehydration may make you feel weak and it may be harder for you to cope with the sensations.

Opioids

Pethidine, Diamorphine, Meptid and Remifentanyl – they might sound like the Four Horsewomen of the Apocalypse, but for some they are knights in shining armour and represent a new dawn. All four drugs are opioids, and they work, not by actually numbing any of your pain receptors, but simply by making you 'out of it' so that you don't experience the pain in the same way. Pethidine, Diamorphine and Meptid are administered via injection in the thigh and in some cases they can be prescribed in advance for a home birth. Remifentanyl comes via an infusion that can only be given by an anaesthetist, so you can't have it at home or in an MLU. One advantage of opioids is that you can get some rest if your labour is long, but bear in mind that if you don't like the feeling they bring, you will have no choice but to wait for it to wear off (except in the case of Remifentanyl; the drip can be turned off and it wears off fairly quickly). Be aware that all four of the opioids cross the placenta and that, the nearer to actual delivery you are given them, the more likely you are to notice an effect in your baby: they may be drowsy, slower to breathe, and breastfeeding may be harder to establish.

Paracetamol

Some women take paracetamol in early labour, and indeed midwives often advise it. It's probably harmless, but you might like to think carefully about how helpful it might actually be, since paracetamol is known to inhibit prostaglandin synthesis. One midwife has called for an investigation into whether paracetamol use in early labour might cause longer and slower latent phases, or even be the cause of 'failure to progress'. More research is needed, but meanwhile, unless you really think it's going to help, it might be best avoided.

Queen

If you ever had any ambitions for diva status, being in labour brings you a golden ticket. You really are the star of this show, so don't be afraid to behave like one, and put as many unreasonable 'riders' in your birth plan as you wish. If you only want red M&Ms in your dressing room, now is the time to say so. Asserting yourself, knowing your rights and being demanding is not only perfectly reasonable when you're birthing a brand new person, but it will also make you feel stronger and more in control, which can have real benefits in the white heat of contractions. How you are treated will directly affect how you feel and how you cope. And make the most of it: once the birth is over your royal status will be well and truly usurped by the one Sigmund Freud so aptly referred to as 'His Majesty The Baby'.

Reframing

Ask yourself – if I'd paid fifty quid for a pill that made me feel this way, would I be enjoying it more? Or – if these sensations were occurring during an intense lovemaking session, how would I be experiencing them? This is 'reframing': seeing the same experience, but through a different lens or frame. So think, 'The next contraction I will reframe as an orgasm'. When it comes, moan, rock and 'pretend' it's gorgeous. The power of your mind may surprise you. (More on page 141.)

Self-Belief

Do you really think you can do this? Have you prepared? Are you a tough cookie? Of course you do, of course you have, and of course you are, so please, believe in yourself. Researchers have actually found that women who go into labour feeling confident are more able to cope. The phrase, 'She believed she could, so she did', might be an overstatement: in labour, as in life, there are no guarantees. But it is true to say that your body knows what to do, so follow its lead and know that, while it may be tough, you can hack it.

Tens Machine

This is a small battery-operated device with little pads that you stick on your sacrum (lower back), where they deliver electrical impulses that feel like tingling sensations. You hold the control unit yourself and decide when to send the impulses and how strong they should be. The TENS is said to work by stimulating endorphins and by reducing the number of pain signals sent to the brain by the spinal cord. You can buy or hire a TENS machine. Some women love them; others don't want to be wired up to a gadget.

Urinate

Have a wee as often as you can because if you let your bladder get full this can cause not only a more painful labour, but also make birth more difficult. If you really can't wee you may need a catheter. So right from the onset of labour, try to keep using the loo. In the throes of labour this can be a tough trip: one of the secret joys of water birth is that you can wee in the pool.

Vocalising

The voice is a natural form of pain relief and release. Anyone who has ever stepped on a piece of Lego in a sleeping child's bedroom will explain this phenomenon to you quite clearly; shouting, roaring, swearing and hollering are necessary and useful responses to pain. In labour you can harness this idea, but use your voice effectively – you don't want to waste energy. Moaning, chanting, singing or even mooing like a cow can feel absolutely brilliant. Keeping your noises low and sexy is generally more helpful than screaming or wailing, but do what feels right.

Water

Wallow in a deep pool, stand under a hot power shower, have your birth partner pour warm scoops over your back, run the taps or just stand next to a river: labouring women report that all kinds of water can help in all kinds of ways. It's the feminine element, and it's often used to help people and even animals in pain, so it makes sense that it would work for labour. Being in a birth pool is widely reported to be bliss. (For more see water birth on page 157.)

Xylophone

OK, so I got a bit stuck on 'X' – but this type of pain relief comes in the form of music, which can of course be played on the xylophone, although most prefer CD or MP3. Your favourite music can uplift you, whether it's something to gyrate to in early labour or a meaningful piece that you have already enjoyed playing to your baby or listening to while visualising your birth. And there is a scientific basis to this: music stimulates areas of the brain, including the hippocampus, and it's widely accepted that it can influence our hormones and our mood. Although, even the scientists agree that *Ring of Fire*, the Beatles' *Help*, and the theme tune from *The Omen* are all best avoided; even the xylophone versions.

Yoga

It's no surprise that pregnancy yoga has become such a 'thing', since the mind-body connection, focus on the breath, and attention to the power of movement that it brings can be just the ticket when it comes to coping with labour pain. Find a class that specialises in yoga for birth preparation, and allow the magic of peaceful, meditative shapes to go to work on your clumsy pregnant bod. In labour you will be able to draw on the techniques you have learnt and use them to help you cope.

Zone

Some call it Labour Land, some the Zone, some speak of a personal bubble. Whatever you choose to call it, at some point in your labour you will withdraw to this place and, once you are there, you will be using many of the tools above and your own resources to cope brilliantly with the rollercoaster ride of labour. All of your attention will be needed. Try to avoid anything that will take you out of the Zone; for example, people you don't feel safe or comfortable with, or interruptions. Being asked questions can also draw you out of this place, so perhaps consider making sure your partner knows your wishes and is prepared to speak for you. Do not fear the Zone; many women love this place and find they feel strong and vital in it.

chapter 4

Watermelons, Bowling Balls and Tooth Extractions:

more about the reality of labour

The idea that childbirth is a massive design-fault is pretty persuasive, isn't it? When you're pregnant, jovial chat about the seemingly impossible feat of sprog-popping can fill your head and echo round endlessly, especially as your bump starts to grow and everyone, even the woman in the frozen veg aisle, sees fit to cheerfully tell you how 'enormous' you are. 'Yes, yes, I am enormous', you think to yourself, 'and this is because a huge headed creature is growing inside of me, and it's got to get out of a neat little hole that has so far only been wide enough for a super-plus tampon or a comparatively small willy.' (Don't say this out loud in the frozen veg aisle, you may cause widespread panic.)

Then another kindly soul will positively guffaw at your mention of birth without high-level pain relief, saying, 'You wouldn't have a tooth out without drugs, wouldya luv?'

The whole concept of giving birth can seem totally unnatural and impossible, but let's pause for a moment, take a breath, and take in some facts.

First of all, the baby's head. A baby's head is not a solid object like a bowling ball or a watermelon. As it moves down the birth canal, the pressure can feel huge, and it's certainly not your average sensation, so perhaps this is why women sometimes use these metaphors to try to convey just what a mind-blowing feeling it is. But in reality, the bones of the baby's head at the time of birth are not hard and unyielding, nor can they damage you. They are soft and moveable, with two soft spots, or fontanelles, which allow your baby's head shape to change as they are being born in a process called 'moulding'. After birth, the bones of the skull will slowly fuse and the soft spots will close over time. All in all a good piece of design and engineering.

The second, and arguably even more impressive piece of intelligent design in the birth process is your amazing vagina. Yes, you probably knew that penises could change shape and expand in often pretty surprising ways, but did you know that your female body possessed similar talents?! As you give birth, and the baby descends, your vagina will get as big as it needs to get to allow the baby a smooth exit, and it's absolutely built to do this in a way that no other part of the body is. So if anybody tells you that giving birth is like pushing a golf ball out of your nostril, it's time to gently enlighten them about the unique and mind-bendingly stretchy qualities of your vag. Well, they started it!

Finally, the tooth removal. If having a baby is in any way a comparable experience to a trip to the dentist – people in white coats, bright lights, painful extractions – then do, please, take every drug on offer. The thing is, it shouldn't be. Your body is designed to give birth to a baby, and in the right circumstances, with the right support, a beautiful hormonal dance will take place within you that will mean that birth will happen at a pace you can cope with and with sensations that may be tough, but manageable. Talk of dentistry implies that birth is essentially something going wrong in the body, when in fact, it's the opposite – it's your body at its healthiest and most vital.

Will there be lots of blood?

People often labour under the misapprehension that childbirth is a bloody, gory affair. 'I wouldn't like to give birth at home,' such people will often say, 'What about all that mess??!!'. These are the kind of comments that make us very, very anxious about birth. 'What the heck did they mean?', we wonder to ourselves when we're seven months pregnant and can't sleep and it's 4am. 'What exactly is going to happen to me? Will it be like a scene from *Alien*?!'

Please let me reassure you that it most certainly will not. Many women in the early stages of labour bake cakes, chat to their midwives, make out with their partners, or take their older kids to the swings. You will look normal; in fact probably better than normal, as you will have the lovely rosy glow of oxytocin, and there won't be any blood.

In the run-up to labour or the early stages, you might lose your mucus plug and this is sometimes called a 'bloody show'. This is just a little jelly-like blob that you might not even notice. It is usually pinkish in colour and there may be a very small amount of blood. Anything more than a spot or two could be a sign that something is wrong and, if you are in any doubt, speak to your midwife.

Often waters will break during labour and this is especially common at transition. It's great to be in the birth pool at this point as this will mean you don't have to pay the situation any real attention. If you're not in the pool, the midwives will be experts in placing towels or 'inco pads' in all the right places. And if your waters break in early labour or before labour starts, you might need to cross your legs and make a sprint for the loo. Again, there shouldn't be any blood at this time, although your waters might have a pinkish tinge. If there is any meconium in your waters, or anything else you feel is unusual, your midwives need to know.

When you actually give birth, there will be a little bit of blood – how much varies from woman to woman. There is also some blood after the baby is born, and during the third stage with the arrival of the placenta. If you tear or have an episiotomy during delivery, then this will bleed slightly. There may also be a small amount of poo (see next page). Again, midwives are adept at keeping you and your bed or floor clean, and you probably won't notice any blood or any other bodily emissions being cleared away as you will be too busy looking in amazement at your baby.

Once you have delivered the placenta, uterine contractions will close off its blood supply and any small amount of bleeding should stop. Any large amounts of blood loss would be considered a sign of a post-partum haemorrhage, and this happens in only around 5 per cent of births.

Once you are settled after the birth, you will need to use maternity pads for your lochia – this is just like an extra heavy period and happens to all women after childbirth, regardless of whether they had a vaginal or a caesarean birth. Lochia will be bright red initially and may have some clots in it. This is usually normal, but it's a good idea to show them to your midwife. After the first few days the lochia will become lighter in flow and may change to brownish red, but you can expect it to continue for at least two weeks and up to six weeks after the birth. Towards the end it may well be fairly light in flow and can be pink or cream. It's important not to use tampons as this can introduce infection, plus it's good to keep an eye on your lochia and report anything you are not sure about to your midwife.

Like your usual menstrual period, it's best to make friends with your lochia, as it's another sign that your wonderful female body has done, and is doing, something amazingly clever.

What about poo? Will I poo myself in labour?

Rumour has it that a baby isn't the only thing that gets squeezed out of an orifice during labour, and if, like most women, you've only ever defecated on your own behind a locked door, you're probably cacking yourself that such rumours are true.

The bad news is, they are. As the saying goes, shit happens. Because of the proximity – of which I'm sure you are aware – of your rectum and vagina, the pressure of the baby's head as it descends will usually cause a very small amount of poo to come out.

But here's the good news. Not only will you literally not give a crap at this point, as you will be more intensely occupied than you have ever been in your life, but your midwife will be positively delighted to see your output, since, as any midwife will tell you, 'Poo is a sure sign the birth is imminent'.

There's more good news. Not only do midwives love to see poo, they're also experts at whisking it away before you or your partner even notice. They even bring a special sieve to water births expressly for this purpose. This is a fact that may alarm you now, but which in future will make you giggle secretly every time you use a colander.

In birth, as in all other areas of life, a sense of humour is helpful. No matter how your baby emerges, it's never going to be your average day. Strange emissions will almost certainly come from your body: you might moo like a cow, or cry hot rivers of tears, or wee in your birth pool, or vomit all over your mother-in-law. All of these things are normal, and nobody will judge you for them, because you are in the midst of doing something extraordinary.

So yes, you will probably poo. I urge you not to worry about this in the run-up to the birth because you certainly won't worry about it or even notice at the time. And once motherhood is upon you, poo will become a much bigger part of your life. You'll become intimately familiar with and totally relaxed about the workings of another human being's bowels, and will probably even develop names for their extraordinary output: 'The Up-The-Backer', 'The Eruption of Ve-Poo-vius', 'The Poonami'. Once you have hosed yourself and your child down after a few of these incidents, you'll be a number one expert in number twos, and realise that, not only is poo a fact of everyday life, you also need the shit to grow the roses.

Does anyone actually enjoy being in labour?

Absolutely they do! Many women find the whole experience completely exhilarating, a combination of the rollercoaster of physical sensations, the hormonal high, and the emotional thrill of feeling new life come through you and out of you into the world. Let's hear from some of these women, in their own words...

'My first baby was born in a vaginal spontaneous hospital birth in what I have come to refer to as a euphoric birth. I loved to discover all those new sensations that my body had never experienced before, and with them discover all its new capabilities. I loved feeling for the first time a very primal side of me taking over and also experiencing a brief awareness of me clicking into place in a long history timeline of women who came before and who will come after. I loved the strength and power I felt and the anticipation towards the end, the utter amazement in seeing my child and the out of this world empowerment and love feelings I had immediately after . But what I love the most is that 15 years later I know my life was changed by that experience and I'm crying writing to you about it.' Jesusa Ricoy Olariaga

'I felt detached from my surroundings, as if in a bubble, and as if nothing and nobody could touch me... It was wonderful. I could feel incredible intensity and powerful sensations throughout my entire being, which I fully embraced, but experienced no 'pain' at all. I felt like a goddess, a warrior, so earthy, sensual and feminine... I lost all sense of time as I was in my own 'zone' and felt so peaceful and calm. And when the time came to birth my baby, I have never felt such strength, focus, power, determination and absolute belief in myself... I never once doubted my ability to birth my baby. I made primal, bestial sounds as I completely surrendered to the process and let go of all my inhibitions. And at that magical moment when my baby's whole body was born, I felt the hugest

sense of relief, awe, elation and pride at what we had both achieved, as well as everything feeling very surreal and almost impossible to take in... And I wanted to do it all over again! Wow!... That is why I have given birth to four beautiful babies!' Marie Molloy

'Giving birth to my third baby was without a doubt the best time of my life. Once I realised things were really happening, I was on such an indescribable high. I'd looked forward to this day for almost 10 months and it was finally here! Every time I felt a contraction I found myself thinking 'Yes!! This is it!!' That's not to say it wasn't very hard work, and definitely painful at times, but it was the most amazing thing I've ever done (and I felt that at the time, not just looking back).

My labour was fast – I didn't have any checks or monitoring, but I'd say I had barely an hour of established labour – and incredibly intense and primal. I laboured mostly alone as I really needed a quiet environment – I loved that I was able to 'tune out' from everyone and everything and just move how I needed to and make whatever noises I needed to. It was instinctive, powerful and incredible.' Sarah Berryman

'Before I gave birth, I could not for the life of me imagine how I would get that child out of my body. People told me it was possible, but I had this feeling that I wasn't up to the challenge. I had an incredibly long labour, and the hospital staff and I sometimes did not see eye to eye. (For example, though the baby's heartrate was steady, they wanted to see more movement, and it didn't really matter to them that I knew he always slept at that time of day and wouldn't be roused for almost anything. They were pushing for induction and I held them at bay long enough to remember that he'd wake up and start dancing whenever we sang Sabbath songs. So my husband blasted my iPod headphones into my belly and baby started boogieing and the hospital folks were satisfied. Phew!). After that I gained a bit of confidence and just focused on the task at hand. When it finally came time to push I was completely ready to trust myself and my body, and out came my son. Holding him in my arms was amazing and a dream come true, but equally exhilarating was the knowledge that I had climbed this mountain, I'd done it! I felt like a rockstar, like if I could accomplish that, I could do anything! PS: the band we played for him while I was in labour is still one of his favourite groups today.' Gwen E.Vere

'Giving birth to my second baby was the best experience of my life. There was no pain during the labour, well nothing more than mild period-type

pain, and the short (15 minute) second stage was totally ecstatic. I felt one with the universe and understood at a very deep level what mystics mean when they say 'all is well'. It wasn't at all what I expected, as my first labour and birth were days of agony and when he shot out of me I thought my clitoris was ripping in half (it wasn't). With my second I was alone in the bath, the midwives hadn't arrived (they didn't realise the birth was so close as I'd had no pain), my mum had taken my toddler out as I found him distracting, and my husband was in the kitchen making toast. I remember looking out the window at the sky and trees and feeling the most incredible wave of bliss, then I felt stinging so I put my hands between my legs and discovered an entire head (although I simply couldn't believe it at first). I called for my husband and he ran in, after some stating of the obvious "OMG the head is out!!" he delivered the body (of which he is very proud). My baby didn't cry and I whispered loving words to him as I brought him up to my chest. For a moment I felt alarm as I wondered if he was breathing, but then I felt this incredible deep intuitive certainty that he would be fine, that indeed the universe is a safe and loving place, and there is never any reason to fear anything. I would love to have that feeling again.' Heidi Hodder

Can birth be orgasmic?

Orgasmic birth. Yes, you heard correctly. Most of us find it a bit baffling to hear those two words in a sentence together, but one survey by the Positive Birth Movement and Channel Mum has found that as many as 6 per cent of women who give birth have this experience.

This certainly challenges our default image of birth, thanks in part to programmes like *One Born*, of a woman, on her back, on a bed, suffering and begging to be rescued from the pain. It's not exactly *Mills and Boon* material.

But birth is part of the sexual cycle; the same areas of the body are involved, and a woman in labour – on all fours, moaning, rocking, eyes closed – doesn't look a million miles off a woman in the throes of sexual pleasure. Maybe it's time we opened our minds to the possibility that birth might be, if not actually orgasmic, at least filled with the same delicious mixture of pleasurable physical sensations we find when we make love?

Remember: expectations can shape reality!

We might be shocked that 6 per cent of women report an orgasmic birth, but perhaps our real shock should be that the numbers are so

Shalome Doran, from Melbourne Australia, experienced an orgasmic birth when her third child was born in 2013

During my third pregnancy, I heard about this phenomenon called 'Orgasmic Birth'. After seeing an ecstatic birth video, I immediately thought 'Yes please! I'll have what she's having'. I watched the *Orgasmic Birth* movie by the amazing Debra Pascali-Bonaro and devoured every pleasurable birth story I could find.

In late 2013, my third baby was born at home. I laboured in the privacy of our bedroom, with low lights, meditative music playing, and my man by my side, squeezing my hips during surges. I felt so intimate and connected to him, much more so than our previous birth experiences. It was like we were birthing this baby together.

It was a fast and furious birth, at just 2.5 hours from start to finish. A quick birth is often an intense birth, and while breathing through my surges there was a definite moment when I thought 'Oh wow, this is either about to get really painful, or I can dig deeper and make it amazing'. I dug deeper and I let go. And I mean, I really let go.

I was on fire – every fibre of my being was engaged and pulsing. Another wave started and I focused on the build-up, breathing deep, surrendering to the intensity, riding, riding, riding and then... throwing my head back, moaning out loud, and letting go. It was the most incredible rush, more sensual than sexual. The sounds emitting from my body were orgasmic. I remember wondering if my man had heard the change in me, if he had picked up on the ecstasy that was pulsing through me. I have never felt more feminine, more goddess-like, more womanly, than in that moment.

This experience blew my mind. It shook up every perception I have ever had of birth, and showed me the magic and beauty that can happen when a woman is able to birth in a familiar environment, with her loved ones (and dedicated midwifery team), and with the self-belief that she is capable of greatness. When I saw and read those stories of orgasmic birth, I immediately believed it was possible for me. It is possible for every woman.

low? We certainly wouldn't be too chuffed if the same percentage of women were having orgasmic sex! We've had the sexual revolution – perhaps we need a birth revolution now? Yes, yes, YES!

People keep telling me that giving birth is the most dangerous thing I'll ever do. Is this even true?

The answer to that question is, it depends. There were times in human history, and there still are places on the planet now, where giving birth carries high risks to mother and baby. Factors that are likely to make birth dangerous include:

- Poor maternal diet (leading to conditions like rickets that can affect the shape of the pelvis, or smaller, less healthy babies at birth)
- Poor maternal healthcare (low levels of care for mum and unborn baby; potential problems not spotted in advance)
- Early motherhood (giving birth in adolescence carries higher risks to mother and baby and is more common in developing countries)
- Poor understanding of hygiene (in the 19th century, over half of deaths in childbirth were caused by 'child bed fever', a direct result of doctors not washing their hands)
- Low-skilled attendants (lack of training, lack of knowledge of how to predict problems and deal with them, botched interventions)
- Lack of access to hospital (often due to geography – giving birth in areas where transfer to hospital is long or even impossible)

So when people say things like, 'Home birth doesn't sound safe to me. People die in childbirth in Africa you know!', they are ignoring a lot of these factors, which affect women in some parts of the world, but – very luckily for us – are not on our list of concerns.

If you are giving birth in the 21st-century western world, with full access to first-class healthcare and a wide and healthy diet, then giving birth is actually incredibly safe, for both you and your baby.

A large-scale study called the Birthplace study, published by the University of Oxford in 2011, found that, **'Giving birth is generally very safe. Overall for low-risk women the risk of adverse outcomes was low at 4.3 events per 1000 births.'** ('Adverse outcomes' refers to very serious events such as intrapartum stillbirth, early neonatal death, neonatal encephalopathy, meconium aspiration syndrome, and specified birth-related injuries including brachial plexus injury.)

The Birthplace study looked at the safety of different places of birth (hence the name). The results were surprising to many. In particular, there was strong evidence that choosing to give birth at home is a safe choice to make, particularly for mums who have had at least one baby before. (You can read more about the Birthplace study in the Positive Home Birth chapter).

The Birthplace study also tells us how important it is – and how lucky women in countries like the UK are – to have a 'safety net'. Part of what makes home birth a safe choice in the UK, as well as our first-class midwifery care, is the fact that we have a maternity care system that offers 'back-up' and a quick transfer in the case of an emergency, and offers options to women who have complications and risk factors in their pregnancy or birth.

You might perhaps think that, if we have first-class hospital maternity services, the safest choice would be to automatically plan to give birth there. However, it's really important to remember that birth will not unfold in the exact same way for each woman, no matter where or how she gives birth – it is influenced by the external circumstances. The same woman can give birth in a remote part of Africa, an American hospital, a busy London obstetric unit, a homely birth centre in Holland or her living room floor in Yorkshire, and have very different levels of safety, very different levels of intervention, a very different birth experience and a very different outcome.

So, having the right birth environment (familiar, cosy, quiet, dimly lit) will help improve birth safety. And so will having accessible medical back-up. It is not one versus the other in a big Tealights versus Forceps battle. We need both.

If we have both, then birth is very safe. (For more on this see Evidence-based birth choices on page 148 and What if... I am 'high risk' on page 185.)

❧ chapter 5 ❧

The Choice is Yours

In the next chapter, I'm going to take you through, step by step, everything you need to know to build the ultimate birth plan. But before I do, there are two fundamental facts about having a baby that I want you to take on board. Think of them as two giant steel beams that underpin the whole of the rest of this book and everything in it.

Steel beam #1: You have a choice

Brace yourself for a shocking revelation: in every single pregnancy and birth situation, you have a choice. The end. It really is that simple. What happens to you, your body and your baby in pregnancy, labour and birth, is completely, totally and utterly, Up. To. You.

It's rather extraordinary, when you think about it, that this even needs saying. It's hard to think of another scenario or area of life where the fact that a woman has a choice needs to be made abundantly clear. Your boss cannot tell you that you are not allowed a break or that you can't drink water during your working day. Your husband can't prevent you from going down the pub with your friends or insist that you have sex with him when you totally don't feel like it. These situations would be at best laughable, and at worst, worthy of a court case. In most areas of life, we have a fairly strong sense of our autonomy, and of our rights.

But in the birth room, somehow, we are still in a bit of a Twilight Sleep. We pepper our birth stories with phrases like, 'They wouldn't let me...' or 'I was not allowed'. We follow orders without question. It's hard to know why. Perhaps it's a bit of 'white coat syndrome'. Maybe we trust the docs more than we trust our bodies. Or could there be, dare I say it, a whiff of patriarchy in the air, as we hop up on the bed like good little girls who don't fuss and do as we are told?

Whatever the reason, the total loss of women's power in the birth room can sometimes really stink, and I want to make sure it doesn't happen to you. Of course, I hope that, throughout your pregnancy, labour and birth, you're surrounded by fantastic and supportive professionals, who talk you through all of your options, and encourage you to feel you are in the driving seat when it comes to making informed choices that feel just right for you.

And there might be times when you positively want to place yourself in their hands, if your labour really isn't unfolding as it should, or if you feel or are told that something is definitely not right and you need medical help. At these moments, most women readily let the experts around them take the reins, and in the midst of crisis, their assistance is gratefully received and usually of stellar quality.

But there are many, many more choices to be made in pregnancy and birth that are not life or death decisions, and I want to encourage you to take an active interest, not only in the finer details of these choices, but also in your right to be informed, and then choose to accept or decline what is being offered to you. Let's think of some examples. When you are in labour, will you allow a midwife to examine your dilation at regular intervals? If you go overdue, do you want to have a 'sweep'? At what stage, if any, will you accept induction? Do you want a VBAC, and if so, would you like to be at home? If your baby is breech, do you want to try ECV? And will you say yay or nay to vitamin K?

The choices are literally endless, and I really can't tell you what to do, although at times you may wish somebody would. I can only tell you to do your homework, and insist that your healthcare professionals inform you about the latest guidelines and evidence, and the benefits and risks of every intervention.

Above all, know that, while the choice may be complex, it is entirely yours to make. Your birth is much more likely to feel positive if you take an active rather than a passive role in what happens to you.

Steel beam #2:
You have human rights in childbirth

Not only do you have a choice about everything that happens to you in birth, but – and this may be an even bigger shock – you have human rights. Human rights? In childbirth? This notion often doesn't quite compute: we're just not used to these two particular concepts being anywhere near each other. But as a pregnant woman, you certainly do have rights. You have a voice in childbirth, you have autonomy over your own body and what happens to it, and these rights, just like all other human rights, are enshrined in law.

In 2010 a landmark case known as Ternovsky vs Hungary in the European Court of Human Rights ruled that every woman has the right to give birth where and how she chooses.

Furthermore, just as you have the right to accept or decline any medical intervention or treatment when you are not pregnant, you keep this same right when you are pregnant or in labour.

In the UK, the law is agreed that the baby in the womb doesn't have any rights until the moment they are born. This might sound harsh, but actually it's quite an effective way of keeping things very 'black and white' and protecting the rights of the woman carrying the child. In countries where the unborn child has rights, difficult situations can arise where the freedom of the mother is compromised, for example, by enforced caesarean sections.

Under UK law, as long as you have mental capacity you cannot be forced to accept any treatment, even if it that treatment is deemed to be in the interest of your unborn child.

In reality, of course, it's extremely unlikely that any pregnant woman would decline a treatment that she was told was important to hers or her baby's welfare. However, just knowing that you do have rights can bring a welcome shift to the power dynamic of the birth room: the right to choose is always yours, regardless of whether or not you decide to exercise that right.

It's also interesting to consider that you do have the right to say no to the many non-emergency interventions that you will be offered in pregnancy and birth. For example, you don't have to have ultrasound scans, or membrane sweeps to start your labour, or vaginal exams to check your dilation.

You may be entirely happy to have all of these things, but it's vital to remember that it's your choice and yours alone.

To make a choice, you need to be fully informed. Why is this intervention helpful or necessary? What are the benefits, and what are the risks? What do the NICE guidelines say about this intervention? What evidence is available to support it? And is this intervention offered or recommended to all pregnant women in the same situation, nationwide? Or is this specific to the policy of this particular hospital, or consultant?

Be a pest. Ask these questions. You are entitled to be fully informed about all of your options at every stage of pregnancy, labour and birth. It is also worth noting that – in the eyes of the law – consent that is not informed is simply not valid. In other words, if you don't fully understand what you are agreeing to, your consent is meaningless.

Remember this, if you remember nothing else from this chapter: You are allowed. You are allowed to say yes or no to any of the options offered to you. You have the full right to be the key decision-maker in what happens to you and your body and your baby during labour and birth, and this is supported by law.

There might be some choices that you are absolutely happy to agree to, and others that you want to say no to. This is not an all or nothing situation, nor is it about starting a war with your caregivers – indeed, working in partnership with your caregivers is the absolute best option for developing a safe and personalised care plan that feels right for you. However, it's vital that all women become aware of their human rights in childbirth, in particular with regard to their own bodily autonomy, and that they have the confidence to exercise those rights, should they so wish.

Rights in birth are not just about consent, they are also about the way you deserve to be treated. Research – and the stories women tell about their births – shows that being treated with dignity, listened to and respected during your birth experience means you are more likely to feel positive about it afterwards, regardless of the place or mode of delivery.

Sometimes challenging hospital protocol or opting out of any aspect of your standard maternity care can be difficult. If you need further support or a place to discuss your choices, try your Supervisor of Midwives, Birthrights, AIMS or the Positive Birth Movement.

Human Rights in Childbirth

Rebecca Schiller, founder and CEO of Birthrights, and author of *Why Human Rights in Childbirth Matter*, talks us through the basics of our human rights in birth

You may not feel like it at times, but you are the same rational, adult human you were before you took the job of incubator for new life. The idea behind the human rights in childbirth movement is nothing more than that. Human rights principles and the legal framework that makes them powerful insist that you are treated with dignity and respect during pregnancy and birth and are never simply viewed as the means to an end.

All public bodies and servants (like hospitals and the doctors and midwives who work in them) must ensure your human rights (as set out in the Human Rights Act 1998 and a series of national, regional and international agreements) are adhered to throughout your pregnancy and birth.

This is good news for you and your baby, as there's a strong relationship between safe, quality care and rights-respecting care. Care that puts you – the pregnant woman – at its heart is better for everyone.

Remember:

☀ You have a right to receive safe maternity care that's appropriate to your needs.

☀ You have the right to privacy and confidentiality.

☀ You have the right to equality and freedom from discrimination.

☀ You have a right to bodily autonomy during pregnancy and birth. Whatever the situation, whatever the intervention, you must be asked for your consent to any procedure and you always have the right to say 'no'.

※ Those caring for you must ensure they explain risks and benefits in an unbiased way that you can understand. They mustn't only give you generic leaflets or one-sided information, but must adapt their discussion to your circumstances and situation.

※ You should be given pain relief when you request it.

※ All reasonable efforts to ensure you can decide where and how you give birth should be made. There shouldn't be blanket bans on certain women having certain kinds of births. Hospitals can have policies and criteria for birth centres and home births, but women outside of these criteria should be enabled to access these birth settings if their requests can reasonably be accommodated.

You can find out more about your rights in pregnancy and birth at **birthrights.org.uk**.

❧ chapter 6 ❧
Planning your birth

Being 'Birthzilla'

Why not having a plan is not a good plan

Have you ever planned a wedding? If so I bet you had a stack of mags, a Pinterest board that creaked under its own weight, and so many lists that you had to make an alphabetical list of your lists. You knew that some of it you couldn't afford, you knew it might rain, and you had a slight unspoken fear that, if you let yourself get any more Bridezilla, it might not actually happen at all, but my God you had your lists, and you were on it.

Or maybe you're not that bothered about weddings, but you've got a clear idea how to take your business to the top, get your product on the shelves, or get promoted or voted or quoted. You have dreams, you have ambition, you have a plan. Whatever you're aiming for, nobody would question that.

Unless you're pregnant. If you're pregnant, you might sometimes find yourself using a shrugging, light-hearted or hesitant tone, and saying something like, 'Well I want to do things as naturally as possible, but you can't really plan these things so I'll probably just go with the flow'.

Unfortunately, you're probably saying this because you have heard this message repeatedly and begun to accept it as fact against your better judgement. As soon as you're pregnant, at least one person, and usually several, will warn you against making any kind of plan for your birth, because 'Birth is unpredictable'.

Birth is unpredictable. Yes. This is indeed correct. But as I am a grown woman and presumably you are too, let me tell you something you already know. Life is unpredictable. It has an unreliable, fickle, and unstable nature that, quite frankly, completely sucks. Anybody who has got past twenty and been let down, bereaved, jilted, done over or disappointed knows this to be true. It might be fair to say we all have an unspoken motto: 'Have plenty of sparkly and ambitious plans. Accept majority will get pissed on and come to nought.'

But still, grown-up women who know all this are told, 'Don't make a birth plan. You will only end up disappointed'.

This defeatist approach is disempowering. It encourages people who might normally read, research, think hard and make lists of their lists to instead lie back and let the whole birth thing just wash over them. But while 'going with the flow' might feel like a plan in itself, it isn't – it's just being passive and handing over the reins to somebody else.

Of course, in an ideal world, you could argue, we wouldn't need a birth plan. In an ideal world, we'd all have a relationship with our midwife (see page 152) and she'd spend time getting to know us in our pregnancy and coming to a unique understanding of the kind of birth we want. And in an ideal world, you could also argue, women wouldn't need to write in their birth plan that they want things like optimal clamping and skin-to-skin, because they'd get it as standard. But – sorry folks – this is not an ideal world.

It's true that birth is unpredictable, but don't let that fool you into thinking the whole thing is just pot luck. There are elements that you can include in your birth preferences that will maximise your chances of having a positive experience. They won't be a cast-iron guarantee (remember that bit about how life really sucks?) But they will maximise your chances.

Birth plans are not just idyllic wish lists lit by pretty tea-lights and trimmed with home-made bunting. A birth plan is a chance to take a detailed look at the huge number of choices and options available to you, to consider the many ways birth might unfold, and to really make sure your voice is heard in the labour room. Your list of options is endless and worthy of a great deal of time and consideration. I'll cover as many as I can in the pages that follow, and we'll also look at ways you can plan for different scenarios. In other words, ways to build not just Plan A, but Plan B and C as well.

You might hear some people express anxiety about birth plans, with even some birth professionals disliking the word 'plan' and arguing it should be replaced with 'preferences'. But to me this PC-speak just colludes with the social message that pregnant women shouldn't bother trying to take control of their births. Call your plan by the name that feels right for you, but ultimately, don't be afraid to

> 'What's in a name? That which we call a rose
> By any other name would smell as sweet.'
>
> **William Shakespeare,** *Romeo and Juliet*

admit that it's a document that sets out exactly how you want things to be, and that – since you are a fully grown woman – you're likely to have thought through more than one scenario, and be capable of holding it together if your plans have to change.

So make a birth plan, building in your wants and needs for every situation, and let those two big steel beams – CHOICE and RIGHTS – underpin it. Knowing you were in charge of your decisions and that you were listened to and treated with respect will make more difference to the way you feel about your birth afterwards than the actual mode of delivery.

Take time to learn about your options. Make it your pregnancy project, and do not let anyone tell you you're wasting your time. Go with the flow at your peril. Plan for the best case and the worst case scenario. Read. Make lists of lists. If necessary, be Birthzilla.

The Visual Birth Plan (VBP)

Your birth plan is a document for both you and your care providers. It's a way of setting out for yourself the kind of birth you want, and of thinking about what is important to you even if your birth deviates from your hopes. It's also a piece of paper to show your midwives or other professionals to help them be clear about the choices you have made.

Since we live in a busy world, I think the best birth plan for real speed and clarity is an 'Iconographic' or 'Visual' birth plan. Throughout this chapter, you'll see a series of icons to represent different birth choices, and by using them, you can build up a birth plan that will be completely unique to you and your choices (there are samples to get you thinking on pages 79 and 80).

These icons are unique to this book, and if you wish, you can download them for free at **pinterandmartin.com/vbp** and use them to build your own personal VBP. You may also wish to make a more detailed written birth plan to accompany your VBP and there are samples of these later in this chapter.

Let's get started on building your birth plan by working step-by-step through the many questions you'll need to consider. Along the way we'll build up a picture of the kind of birth you really want. We'll also look at other scenarios and at building a clear plan for them as well.

Where do you want to give birth?

There are four main places you can give birth: home, midwife-led unit (MLU), obstetric unit, or the operating theatre. For more information on each place of birth see pages 182 to 217.

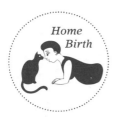
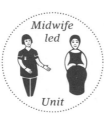
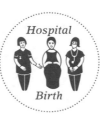
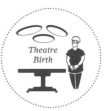

Who do you want to be with you?

(Put this info in a box at the top of your VBP.) It's important to name on your birth plan the people you hope will be supporting you. Your partner, your doula, your mum, your friend. Think carefully about who you want to bring into your birth space. Your mother-in-law may be keen as mustard, but she might make you feel uncomfortable and make it hard for you to get in the necessary 'zone'. Likewise your BFF might be the most fantastic woman on earth, but if she's never had a baby and is totally terrified, that energy might have a negative impact on you. Try to surround yourself with people who understand you and the kind of birth you want, and who can bring a really calm, helpful presence to your birth room. By the same token, be clear in this area of your birth plan if there is anyone you do not wish to be allowed into your birth room, whether this is someone from your family, or medical students/student midwives.

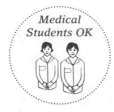
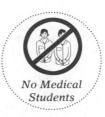

Birth Plan: Charlotte and Martin
Central Hospital, Blackley

Only Charlotte and Martin, and preferably just one midwife in the birth room.

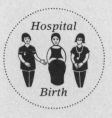

Hospital Birth

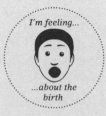

I'm feeling... ...about the birth

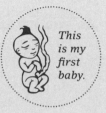

This is my first baby.

Quiet Please No Chatting

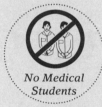

No Medical Students

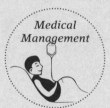

Medical Management

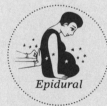

Epidural

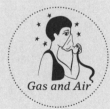

Gas and Air

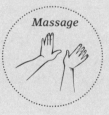

Massage

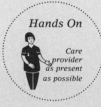

Hands On Care provider as present as possible

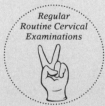

Regular Routine Cervical Examinations

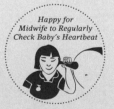

Happy for Midwife to Regularly Check Baby's Heartbeat

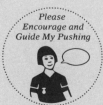

Please Encourage and Guide My Pushing

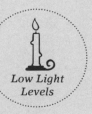

Low Light Levels

Delayed
Active Management

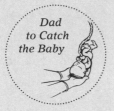

*Dad
to Catch
the Baby*

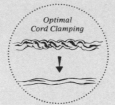

*Optimal
Cord Clamping*

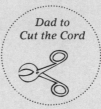

*Dad to
Cut the Cord*

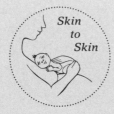

*Skin
to
Skin*

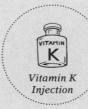

*Vitamin K
Injection*

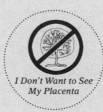

*I Don't Want to See
My Placenta*

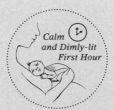

*Calm
and Dimly-lit
First Hour*

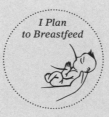

*I Plan
to Breastfeed*

Birth Plan: Maria and Tom
Central Hospital, Blackley

We've laid out the kind of birth we really want in this plan. However, we hope to work with our caregivers as a team and are flexible and open minded. We will have Maria's mum and a doula in our birth space with us.

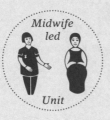

Midwife led Unit

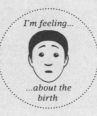

I'm feeling... ...about the birth

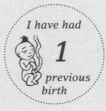

I have had 1 previous birth

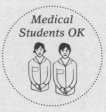

Medical Students OK

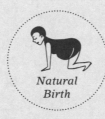

Natural Birth

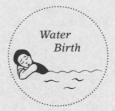

Water Birth

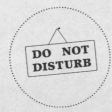

DO NOT DISTURB

Don't Say Contractions / Please Say Surges

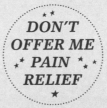

DON'T OFFER ME PAIN RELIEF

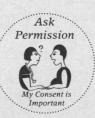

Ask Permission / My Consent is Important

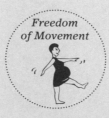

Freedom of Movement

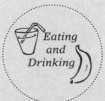

Eating and Drinking

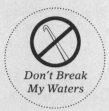

Don't Break
My Waters

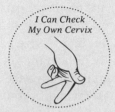

I Can Check
My Own Cervix

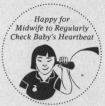

Happy for
Midwife to Regularly
Check Baby's Heartbeat

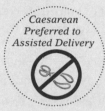

Caesarean
Preferred to
Assisted Delivery

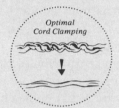

Optimal
Cord Clamping

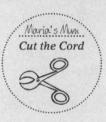

Maria's Mum
Cut the Cord

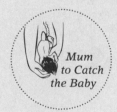

Mum
to Catch
the Baby

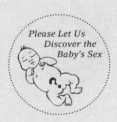

Please Let Us
Discover the
Baby's Sex

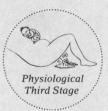

Physiological
Third Stage

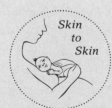

Skin
to
Skin

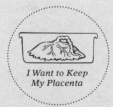

I Want to Keep
My Placenta

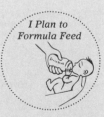

I Plan to
Formula Feed

A bit about you and your history

Use this part of your birth plan to give your care providers a quick overview of you and the kind of birth you want. If you are doing a written birth plan to accompany your VBP, you can go into more detail, but the icons that follow should help give a brief outline of the birth you're hoping for and how you are feeling. I can't think of anyone who wouldn't want to include the icon requesting that their permission be sought for every intervention, but if you have a history of abuse (see page 92), this might be especially important to you.

It's true that you might not know in advance exactly what you are going to want in labour, especially if this is your first baby. You might think you'll want to do the whole thing in a room by yourself, but end up spending most of your labour nose-to-nose with a midwife who you vow will be top of your Christmas list for the rest of your life. You might think you've got a low pain threshold, and then discover on the day you have the soul of a Samurai.

Lay out in your plan what you think you're going to want, then be prepared to change tack on some aspects (you might say no to student midwives, but then meet one and really click with her), and stick to others (like optimal cord clamping) like superglue.

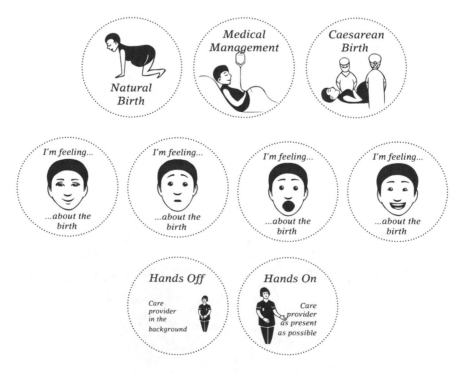

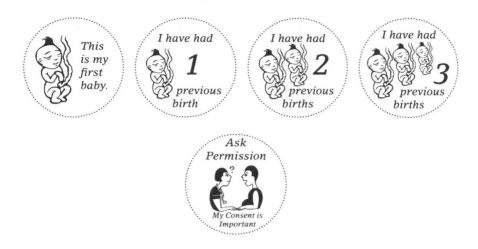

Any other special requirements?

If you or your birth partner have a disability that you think it might be helpful for professionals to be aware of, if you are giving birth in a part of the world where the language spoken is not your first language and therefore need an interpreter, or if you have any religious, spiritual or cultural requirements that your caregivers need to know about, put this information near the top of your plan.

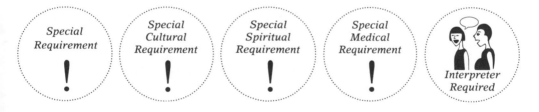

What kind of birth environment do you want?

Listen up, because this bit is vital: the environment you give birth in is going to have a direct impact on your physical and emotional experience of birth, and even on the way that your labour and birth unfolds. You need to give birth in a place and an environment that makes you feel safe, and allows you to produce oxytocin (see page 128). This will not be the same place or environment for every woman – we are all different!

Producing oxytocin is important for bonding and breastfeeding, and for your overall feeling of wellbeing, so it should be a consideration for every woman, regardless of whether she wants a home birth or a caesarean. It's also vital to remember that oxytocin production needs to keep going as you meet and feed your baby too, so the birth environment needs to be kept calm and dim for the Hour of Power too (see page 102).

Basically, it's essential to remember that we are all mammals, and mammals have very similar criteria for their birth space: dark, quiet, private, undisturbed. Wherever you decide to give birth, you need to make sure you create an environment that ticks these boxes. If you choose hospital for your place of birth, you may have to work a bit harder at this, for example by taking in comforting and homely possessions, by rearranging the furniture, or by making sure the lights are kept low or dimmed. Your partner or doula may have to take charge of making sure this happens for you, by becoming your 'Guardian of Oxytocin' (see page 130).

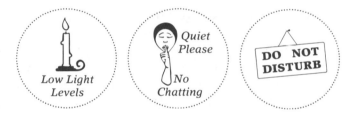

Mind your language! Considering the words we use

Some people like to change the language they use around childbirth, and ask that others who come into their birth space do so too. This is because of the connection between mind and body, and the acknowledgement that how we talk and think can affect what our bodies actually 'do' (or refuse to do). (For more on the mind body connection see page 136).

Some of the words that people like to challenge or replace include:

Contractions: some argue that the very word makes them sound worse than they are; others think it's a pretty accurate description. Ina May Gaskin (see page 169) uses the word 'rushes'. Others like 'tightening', 'expansion' or 'surge'.

Pain: some people try to speak in terms of 'sensations' or 'pressure' rather than 'pain'. These sensations might be 'powerful' or 'strong'.

Push: We all associate this word with birth, but some argue this comes from managed birth where women – often numb from an epidural – are given instructions from outsiders on what to do and when. Some say you don't need to push at all, anyway (see page 98). Alternatives are 'breathe baby out', or 'bear down'.

Delivery: If you read birth stories in the press, you'll often hear how amazing doctors, burly paramedics, or even heroic dads 'deliver' babies all the time! However, as you are about to discover, there's only one person who can deliver a baby, and that's you (although somebody else may 'catch' it, see page 104). And while we're at it, let's drop 'deliver' completely. Pizzas are delivered. Babies? Babies are born!

There are a few other real stinkers that get used. You might be told that you are 'only 3 centimetres dilated'. Well thanks! That makes it sound like you've hardly bothered, cheers for that. As does 'failure to progress', used when the Cracking On Phase (see page 30) isn't perceived to be cracking on fast enough. Women going for a VBAC get to have a 'trial of scar' (will there be a judge in a wig?), and if your midwife is unenlightened, she may refer to you as, 'my lady in room 6' (you don't belong to her, do you?!) or worse still, tell you you're a 'good girl' (very St Trinian's – and definitely your cue to be naughty).

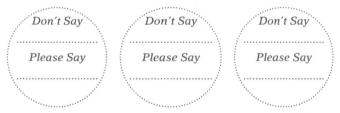

Don't Say

Please Say

Don't Say

Please Say

Don't Say

Please Say

Words matter: don't offer me pain relief!

Some women find even being offered pain relief in labour undermines their confidence in themselves. However well-meaning, being asked, 'Would you like some gas?' or, 'Are you sure you don't want an epidural?', can carry the unspoken message: 'You don't look like you're coping to me'.

Women who want to give birth naturally or without drugs often benefit from putting in their birth plan that they don't want to be offered pain relief. This doesn't mean that they won't even consider having pain relief! It just means that if they want it, they'll ask for it.

What about pain relief?

Choosing the kind of pain relief you want in advance is a bit like booking the restaurants you're going to eat in on holiday before you get there. It's good to have some thoughts about the options, and do your homework, but also good to keep an open mind. In your thoughts about 'pain relief', give some consideration too to the other coping mechanisms and means of self-comfort that you have at your disposal. Think also about ways of maintaining and promoting your strength, for example by taking regular food and drink, or by visualisation or hypnobirthing. (For more suggestions see chapter 3.)

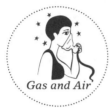
Gas and Air

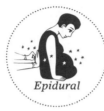
Epidural

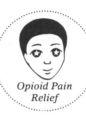
Opioid Pain Relief

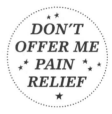
DON'T OFFER ME PAIN RELIEF

Other comfort measures

Some of these elements of your birth plan are really just for your own reference. You would hope, for example, that if you want to eat or drink in labour this will not be up for debate (unless you are on the trolley headed for a caesarean under general anaesthetic, in which case a flapjack is likely to be the last thing on your mind). However, different hospitals in different geographical areas have different policies and protocols, so, as I will keep repeating throughout this chapter, don't make any assumptions. If any aspect is particularly important to you, discuss it with your care providers in advance.

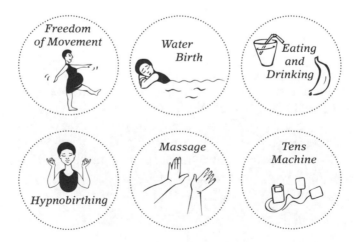

Do you want your labour to be induced?

If you, like many women, find that your due date comes and goes and nothing happens, you will almost certainly be offered the option of induction. As you prepare for your birth it's a good idea to consider whether you will be happy to be induced if you go overdue, or if you would prefer to wait for labour to begin spontaneously. (For more on this see What if... I go overdue? on page 218.)

Do you want your labour to be augmented?

You might also like to consider if you want your labour to be 'augmented' in any way. For example, if it's felt that your labour is progressing more slowly than is thought to be ideal, then it might be suggested that your waters are broken for you (known as artificial rupture of membranes or ARM), or, if your waters have already broken or been broken and still nothing is happening, that you are given drugs to speed up or 'augment' your progress.

Having your waters broken (ARM)

Please know that this should never happen without your express permission. This permission should be sought before any vaginal examination commences and you should be fully informed of what the procedure will entail and what the risks and benefits of it are, in order that you may decline or consent. When considering ARM (Artificial Rupture of Membranes) you may like to note that:

• ARM should not be used routinely, but only if there is concern over the progress of your labour
• it is not proven to be effective in shortening labour
• it can make labour contractions more painful
• it can make you feel like the normal course of your labour has been disturbed
• it increases the need for caesarean
• it increases the likelihood of foetal distress

Drugs to augment labour

If your waters have already broken, or been broken, another way to get labour moving is to give you a drip of synthetic oxytocin or 'syntocinon'. Some hospitals will now offer prostaglandin gel or pessary before the drip, which may be a gentler augmentation and will allow you to stay more mobile. Once you are on a syntocinon drip, your freedom of movement will be restricted and you will need to

Top Tips for Progress 'Failures'

OK, so with your school years far behind you, you didn't think you'd get marked FAIL ever again, right?! Wrong! In labour, this word is often oh-so-kindly used to describe a woman whose labour is not moving fast enough according to the folk who decide on the appropriate speed of the average uterus. Such women, and you may be one of them, will be delighted to discover the term 'Failure to Progress' written on their maternity notes. Great. Just what you need to hear when you've spent 36 hours breathing, chanting and generally feeling like you're nailing it.

If Failure to Progress pays a visit to your birth experience, this could be because your baby is not in a great position (see page 133), or there may not be any obvious explanation. You will almost certainly be offered medical augmentation, but before you make a choice about that, there are a few other ideas you may like to try.

- **Think mammal.** Is the room dark or dimly lit? Do you feel safe? Are you warm enough? Is there anyone in the room who does not need to be there or who, worse still, is annoying you? Is the room quiet? Think about this in advance with your partner, as being a Guardian of Oxytocin (see page 130) is a role they can help with.
- **Gimme some lovin'.** If your birth environment gets a 10 out of 10, try other ways of getting the oxytocin flowing. Snog, smooch, stimulate your nipples or clitoris, or even orgasm if you feel like it. Get rid of the midwives first, perhaps?
- **Move.** Change position. Walk. Get on a birth ball. Get on all fours. Get off the bed. Try anything to change the energy in your body, even if you have to leave the labour room.
- **Eat and drink.** Low energy has a lot to answer for in labour. It's so important to keep your intake of fluids and easy grazing foods up.
- **Acupuncture or acupressure.** You can have an acupuncturist on speed dial as part of your birth team, or you might be lucky enough to be in a hospital that provides one. You can also get your partner to give you acupressure or do it yourself – google 'acupressure for labour' to find points to gently stimulate.
- **Free your mind (and the rest will follow).** Make sure there are no thoughts or feelings that might be holding you back. Talk to your partner or midwife. Voice your fears out loud. Cry. This psychological release may have a corresponding effect on your body.

have regular VEs and CTG monitoring to check how your body and your baby are responding to the drug. Like ARM, having your labour augmented in this way may mean it is more uncomfortable for you, and makes further interventions more likely.

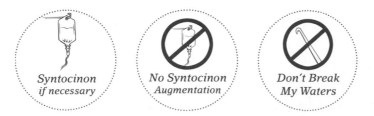

Syntocinon if necessary   *No Syntocinon Augmentation*   *Don't Break My Waters*

Do you want to have routine vaginal exams (VEs) to assess your dilation?

Vaginal, or cervical examinations as they are also known – when a midwife, or sometimes a doctor, inserts fingers into your vagina and checks how dilated you are – are one of those things that come as standard in labour, unless you request otherwise. Usual policy is to check your dilation every four hours even if there are no concerns about you, your baby, or your progress. Hopefully, if you've been paying attention to this book, you'll know by now that you have the right to accept or decline any intervention in pregnancy or labour that you don't want, and the routine cervical exam is one area where many women are choosing to say, 'Thanks, but no thanks'. Some women feel that the exams are uncomfortable and distract them from the 'zone' of 'Labour Land'. Often, to have an exam, you will be asked to get out of the birth pool if you are in one, or lie on the bed even if you are labouring actively. You can see that this could be a most unwelcome distraction and could, to borrow a term from golf, completely put you off your stroke. Other women dislike the exams because of the risk of infection and the risk that your waters will get accidentally broken by the midwife's fingers. Many argue that if labour is 'cracking on', it will probably be obvious to you and all around you, so the disruption of the checks is unnecessary. However, if you feel curious about your dilation you can always ask for a quick check.

You may also like to consider the option of 'DIY'. If you want to feel how things are progressing, there is nothing to stop you from using your own fingers to feel how things are changing inside you, and many women who do this report that it can be extraordinarily joyful and encouraging to feel the top of their baby's head for the very first time! Some also get their husbands or partners to check – and this is also 'allowed'!

Giving birth as a survivor of abuse

Your body, like a beautiful landscape, or, if you prefer, an overgrown garden, has edges. It has borders. It has places where it stops, and the rest of the world begins. You are the undisputed queen of this land, and others do not have the right to cross your boundaries or walk on your soil without your express permission. This is bodily autonomy.

It's important to know that you have full autonomy over your body and what happens to it in pregnancy and birth, just as you do in any other circumstance of life. You cannot be made to give up a kidney, have a tooth extracted or give blood, for example, without first being informed about what will happen, told of any risks, and giving your full permission. Anything that happens to you in labour and birth is no different.

This might be particularly helpful for you to know if you have experienced abuse in the past. Any kind of abuse, whether it happens during your childhood or as an adult, or whether it is physical, sexual or emotional, involves a 'trespass' across the border-lines, an invasion of your personal space to which you very much do not consent.

Childbirth can often awaken memories of these experiences for women, and it is therefore really important that, if you are a survivor of abuse, midwives and doctors treat you with dignity and respect and most importantly understand that 'stop means stop' and 'no means no'.

Even with the most respectful caregivers, giving birth can sometimes trigger very difficult feelings for survivors. You might find that the physical feelings involved in labour upset you, or that you really dislike the loss of control or 'surrender' that comes with having a baby.

What can you do?

- Seek specialist support: find a counsellor, doula or midwife who is trained to understand the issues around giving birth as a survivor of abuse. They will be able to support you and understand you as you prepare to give birth.
- Some women who have survived abuse like to tell their care providers about this, ask their partner or doula to do so, or state this in their birth plan, so that professionals are aware and can be

extremely sensitive. However, it can be very difficult to open up to relative strangers about your past experiences and there should be no pressure on you to do so.

- Regardless of whether or not you want to overtly state that you are an abuse survivor, you can still put clear instructions in your birth plan about your wishes. For example, you may want to put in writing that you wish to be clearly asked for your consent before all procedures, or that you do not wish to have any VEs (vaginal examinations, see page 91).

- Some survivors of abuse find it helpful to get more information about what birth is like, and if you are reading this book you are probably one of them. Reading empowering birth stories or watching films of beautiful, gentle births can both allay your fears and help make the distinction between the difficult events that happened in your past, and the experience of childbirth.

I dream of a day when there is a better awareness of this issue. In the meantime, know that part of the movement towards more respect for bodily autonomy in the birth room comes from you. Make sure both you and your birth partner fully understand your rights in the birth room and do not hesitate to assert them. Whatever your personal history, remember that you are queen of your bodily landscape.

For those who do wish to tell their care providers about this aspect of their history, we've made a choice of three icons for Survivor of Abuse, but don't feel you have to use any of them unless you want to. An alternative is the Ask Permission icon from page 85.

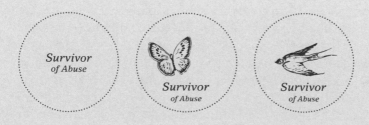

If you don't want any routine cervical checks in labour, it's a really good idea to discuss this with your midwives in advance. If you feel it necessary, get your lead midwife to sign your birth plan to say they have approved this or any other decision you feel may be disputed on the day. There are some occasions where the checks are more than just 'routine' and may be considered necessary by your care providers; for example, if you are undergoing a medical induction, or if there are concerns about the length of your labour. There are other occasions where you may be told you 'need' to have a check, for example, 'If you want to get in the pool we need to know how dilated you are first'. It's important to note that regardless of the reason, you do have the right to say no to any examination or intervention during your pregnancy and labour. If there are genuine concerns about you or your baby, you are probably highly unlikely to decline: however, knowing that you can say no can make all the difference to how you feel about your birth experience, both during and after.

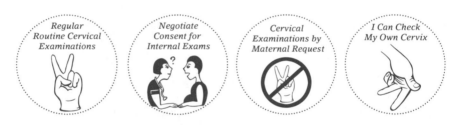

The Bottom Line

Some midwives use other observational skills to assess how quickly or slowly labour is progressing, rather than rely on dilation checks. They will tune in to the sounds and movements you are making, the general 'look and feel' of you, and some midwives even say that women 'smell different' when the birth is imminent! Some midwives will look for a 'purple line', that extends from your – how can I put this delicately... um... I can't – that extends from your anus to the top of your butt crack when you are fully dilated. Research has shown that around 70 to 80 per cent of women get this line, which is caused by the pressure of the baby's head as it descends. As a rough guide, the longer the line extends, the more dilated you are, with the line reaching the top of your crack when you're fully dilated (10cm). The line shows up in most women when they are around 3–4cm, looks most visible around 8cm, and tends to fade again at full dilation. Worth looking out for!

Other kinds of monitoring in labour

As well as checking your dilation every four hours, your midwives will want to 'listen in' to your baby's heartbeat during your labour. This is because sometimes, but very rarely, the stress of the labour itself can have a negative impact on your baby. If the midwives and doctors have a concern about your baby's welfare, they may want to take action such as further monitoring or assessment, and if their concern continues, they may suggest a caesarean birth.

There are several ways that your baby's heartbeat and wellbeing can be monitored during labour.

Pinard, Doppler or Sonicaid
(known as Intermittent Auscultation or IA)

A midwife may listen in to hear your baby's heartbeat using a wooden device that looks like a small trumpet, or a 'Doppler' or 'Sonicaid' that uses ultrasound waves. Standard practice is to listen in every 15 minutes during early labour, and every five minutes in the later stages of labour. Most midwives have 'underwater Dopplers' that can be used if you are having a water birth, and they should be skilled in monitoring you in a sensitive way so that you are not taken out of your 'zone' or disturbed. Some women feel reassured by these regular checks, while others report feeling interrupted or disturbed.

What does the evidence say? The recommended intervals at which the midwife 'listens in' are different in different parts of the world, and it is widely agreed that there is no specific evidence on which to base the regularity of this kind of monitoring. In fact, the practice of listening in at agreed intervals of say, every 15 minutes, is based on 'custom and practice' rather than evidence, according to the Royal College of Midwives. Some argue that the monitoring could be less frequent and still pick up any abnormalities in plenty of time, but there does not seem to be any robust evidence to offer a suggestion of how frequent is frequent enough. As always, you can decide to be monitored less frequently or not at all if you so wish, just as you can also decide to have CEFM even if you have no risk factors and there is no concern for your baby.

Continuous Electronic Foetal Monitoring (CEFM)

This way of listening involves straps around your bump that measure your baby's heart rate and your contractions. If you're giving birth in the USA, it's likely you'll be hooked up to the CTG (cardiotocograph) throughout your labour, while in the UK you will only be offered CEFM if there is a concern about you or your baby. This concern could either arise in labour or beforehand, for example if your pregnancy is considered 'high risk' (see page 185). Being on the CTG may mean that you find yourself on a bed with limited mobility, but try to keep moving if you can, as the wires technically shouldn't stop you. Some hospitals have 'wireless' CTG machines, allowing more mobility or even water birth, so it's worth asking, but rumour has it that they can be tricky to operate and that midwives often despair of them.

What does the evidence say? CEFM seems to be the perfect example of our tendency to assume that shiny expensive machines always make things better and safer, when in fact this is not always the case. There is some evidence that CEFM can prevent neonatal seizures. These occur rarely (about 1 in 500 births) and less rarely when CEFM is used, and their possible long-term effects are unknown. Apart from the reduction in seizures, there is no evidence at all of any advantage to CEFM in either low-risk or high-risk women. It does not reduce instances of cerebral palsy, or the chances of a baby dying. It is, however, associated with a significantly increased risk of caesarean section and instrumental delivery. CEFM has also been found to have a high 'false positive' rate of around 60 per cent – this means it could suggest there are problems with your baby when in fact everything is fine. If CEFM is offered to you, be sure to ask your midwives for the specific evidence upon which they are basing their recommendation.

Foetal Scalp Electrode (FSE)
Sometimes simply called the 'clip', this is an ECG monitor that is attached to your baby's head by inserting a small probe into your baby's scalp. Your waters need to have been broken, and the FSE then monitors your baby's heartbeat via a wire that is connected to the CTG machine. It is sometimes used with something called STAN for more detailed readings. This form of monitoring will sometimes be offered if there are problems getting a reading from the CTG.

What does the evidence say? Your baby should not have a FSE if they are less than 34 weeks' gestation or if you have a blood-borne disease or risk factors for clotting. FSE carries risks to your baby of infection and, in rare cases, damage to their skin or face from the procedure. A Cochrane review of the evidence found that using FSE results in less need for Foetal Blood Sampling and fewer surgical births than using CTG alone. However, it had no effect on the rates of caesarean or on the condition of babies at birth.

Foetal Blood Sampling (FBS)
A small sample of your baby's blood is taken from their scalp using a rod with a small blade attached to it, which is inserted into your vagina. This blood is then tested for oxygen levels, carbon dioxide and acid levels, which can give a more accurate picture of your baby's condition than the CTG. Local anaesthetic spray is applied to your baby's head beforehand. Like FSE, you cannot have this procedure if your baby is premature or if you have a blood-borne disease or clotting risk. Some academics have suggested this test is outdated and not fully supported by evidence.

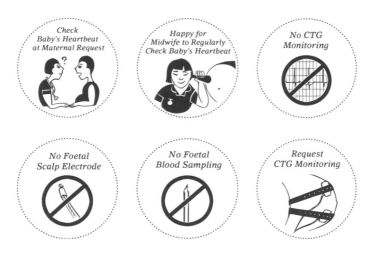

Keep an eye on the monitors
Electronic foetal monitoring is big business. There are approximately 28,000 foetal monitors in more than 3,400 hospitals in the USA, representing an investment of over $700 million dollars.

Source: Evidence Based Birth

What about pushing?

'Push... push... PUSH!' These three little words have become so synonymous with giving birth that it's hard to imagine a baby being born without them. You'd be forgiven for thinking that birth is not even really possible without a small crowd yelling this phrase at your nether regions.

But what if there wasn't any need for this? What if women's bodies could push babies out involuntarily, spontaneously, and without any need for effort, purple faces, bulging eyes or cheerleaders? And what if the three little words we most associated with the moment of birth were not 'Push, push, PUSH', but instead... Foetus Ejection Reflex?

OK. It's not very catchy. It doesn't sound too appealing either, I'll admit. For me it never fails to conjure up an image of the baby sliding out on a little mechanised tray. But don't let this put you off. Because in spite of the rather clunky name, the Foetus Ejection Reflex is one of birth's best kept secrets – and could be the key to quicker, easier and happier births.

When a woman gives birth and the Foetus Ejection Reflex happens, the 'pushing stage' is very quick, usually lasting just a few minutes or less. The woman does not have to make any voluntary effort – her body just takes over and literally ejects or expels the baby in one or two fast contractions. A far cry, perhaps, from the hours of agonised pushing that many women expect as a standard rite of passage into motherhood.

The term Foetus Ejection Reflex (let's call it FER, shall we?), was coined in the 1960s by biologist Niles Newton. Twenty years later, obstetrician Michel Odent took up the term, feeling that it might be key to understanding what is difficult about human birth – and what we could be doing to make it easier.

Odent explains that FER is such a rare phenomenon because we are not providing the birthing environment necessary for it to occur. In order for FER to happen, Odent says, women need to lose control of their 'thinking' brain (the neocortex), which means that the birth needs to be completely undisturbed. Unfortunately, he says, our current approach to birth often expects a woman to give birth in a stark, bright room, observed by strangers. Our modern tendency is also to interfere more and more as the birth becomes imminent, all of which makes FER impossible:

'The reflex does not occur if there is a birth attendant who behaves like a coach, or an observer, or a helper, or a guide, or a "support person"', says Odent in his book *Do We Need Midwives?*. 'The foetus

Experiencing the Foetus Ejection Reflex: Hannah Winbolt Lewis

This birth was different. I didn't really feel a 'second stage' to speak of. I only felt my body begin to heave and lurch: the most tremendously powerful feelings took me over. The best way I can describe it, and this is a phrase I've heard other mothers who have experienced FER use, is that it felt like 'reverse vomiting': that feeling when your body takes over and expulsively forces something out. This sounds unpleasant, but for me it did also feel easy and how nature intended. I'd had two other births – in the first I was on my back being told how to push, holding my breath and straining so hard I broke blood vessels in my face. That was awful. In my second birth I felt under pressure to get in the pool just at the wrong moment, which 'woke me up' and – I believe – caused a tough second stage. But in this third birth, I felt safe and at ease. No one at my birth was an 'outsider'. A friend was there with her breastfeeding baby. My kids were there. It was such an ordinary and extraordinary day all at the same time. I did not feel any need to time, measure or assess my contractions. I just experienced it.

ejection reflex can also be inhibited by eye-to-eye contact or the imposition of a change of environment, as would happen, in our modern world, when a woman is transferred to a delivery room. It is inhibited when the intellect of the labouring woman is stimulated by any rational language, for example if the birth attendant says: "Now you are at complete dilation. It's time to push".'

Odent suggests that women should give birth in a quiet, darkened room with one midwife who keeps her distance, and preferably knits. The reason Odent is such a fan of midwives making woolly hats during labour is because this repetitive exercise gives them something to do and keeps them calm, preventing them from transferring any of their own stress and anxiety to the woman. This then allows the mother to enter what Odent calls a 'quasi-ecstatic state'; any interference will bring her back 'down to earth', preventing the FER and meaning that she will have to consciously push to get her baby out.

As with all advice and information about birth, we probably need to take what we want from FER and leave the rest. We might not experience it, but it's definitely worth questioning whether we need another person to tell us when and how to push. Although some find a professional's guidance at this stage of labour reassuring, many women say that they find the words of an over-enthusiastic midwife intensely annoying or even humiliating: there's nothing like a stranger shouting, 'Push into your bottom!', or even 'Get angry with your baby!' to take some of the romance out of childbirth. It's likely that this practice of coached pushing stems from the use of epidural anaesthesia: if you are numb from the waist down, then delivering your baby really does need to be a team effort. But if you haven't chosen epidural, it might be interesting to listen to your body and follow its lead. Like everything else in this book, it's about choice: if you don't want your midwife's direction, tell them to push, push, push off.

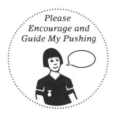

Please Encourage and Guide My Pushing

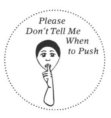

Please Don't Tell Me When to Push

What if I need an assisted delivery?

During your birth, you may be advised that an 'assisted' or 'instrumental' delivery is needed to help your baby to be born. This means that an obstetrician will attend your birth, and guide your baby out using either forceps – which look rather like metal salad servers – or ventouse (or the smaller version called a Kiwi cup), which is a silicone cup that's attached to your baby's head.

You will usually be on a bed with your feet in stirrups (known as the lithotomy position), and will sometimes be taken to theatre. If you have not already had an epidural, you may be offered one, or you may be given local anaesthetic. The doctor may make an episiotomy – a small cut to your perineum – to make your vaginal opening wider. This will need to be repaired with stitches after the birth. Sometimes, the assisted delivery will be unsuccessful, and at this point the next option is a caesarean birth.

Assisted delivery usually happens because of:

- Concerns over the baby's heart rate
- Baby being in an awkward position
- You being tired or exhausted

There are risks to an assisted delivery. These include an increased risk of tearing (see page 229), a higher risk of blood clots, and an increased risk of incontinence after the birth. There is also a risk to the baby of cuts or bruising to the face and head, although these are usually minor and heal within a few days of delivery.

It's hard to say many positive things about assisted delivery. Giving birth with the help of items that would not look out of place in your kitchen is unlikely to be at the top of any woman's wish list, but it happens. If it happens to you, remember:

- Ask questions. Can you have more time? If the reason given for assisted delivery is that you are too tired, can you address this in other ways? Have you eaten and drunk enough? Can you call on any reserves of strength, or are you 'done'? (See BRAIN on page 119.)
- If you are 'done', you might find an assisted delivery is not as bad as you are expecting. Some women report that it's a great relief to have this help to birth their baby, having reached a point where they feel completely happy to accept this intervention.
- If you absolutely don't want an assisted delivery under any circumstances, put in your plan that you would rather have a caesarean. There are, of course, risks associated with a caesarean (see page 207), but you need to balance these with the risks of an assisted delivery, and in particular how it might make you feel during and after if you are really opposed to it.
- If you do decide to have an assisted delivery, keep strong using breathing techniques, meditation, visualisation or hypnobirthing to help you. (See also HEART on page 120.)
- After the birth, take extra care of your perineum. (See box on page 230.)

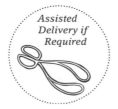
Assisted Delivery if Required

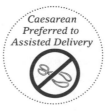
Caesarean Preferred to Assisted Delivery

Lateral thinking, upright birth: Liz Martindale, a consultant obstetrician at Burnley General Hospital in Lancashire, has facilitated several assisted deliveries where, rather than being in stirrups, the mother has been either kneeling on the floor, or in a standing position

'In one of the first of these cases, the woman had had a previous caesarean where she had felt she had no control or influence over the birth process', Liz explains. 'In her birth in our unit, she had been pushing for two hours. She was comfortable standing up and we were able to examine her in that position. A Kiwi cup was used to bring the head to the perineum and then removed. A normal birth was facilitated by the student midwife, with the patient leaning over the bed. She was delighted with her birth experience, particularly the fact that she was able to give birth in her chosen position and felt that she was empowered.

The positive birth experience shows how collaborative working among professionals can push the boundaries when promoting positive birth, resulting in an unusual and satisfying birth. By listening to the woman's fears and empowering her rather than insisting on conventional assisted delivery in lithotomy, a positive birth experience was achieved.

Although safety of mother and baby are paramount, the effect of birth experience should always be considered. By taking a holistic and team approach in this case, we helped redress the previous traumatic birth. The delivery itself was not difficult for the medical staff, but required "lateral thinking". Similar positive births have followed on from this case in our unit.'

The Hour of Power

If you're paying attention, you've probably got the point now that I think preparing and planning for birth is one of the smartest things you'll ever do. But while you might be madly researching your choices and options for every stage of labour, I bet there's one part of having a baby you haven't really thought about: the first hour after birth, a time I call the Hour of Power.

Why do I call it this? Because it's a vital time, when a powerful bond that lasts a lifetime is just beginning. And because it's a time when you are holding your 'prize', earned by the hard work of labour, and hopefully feeling more powerful than you ever have in your life. Birth pioneer Michel Odent says of this time, 'Don't wake the mother'. As hard as it may be, especially in a busy hospital, it's so important that this time is as undisturbed as possible. The Hour of Power belongs to you, your partner and your baby, and no one else.

If you've watched enough *Call the Midwife* you'll probably have a vision of yourself just after birth, sweating and pasty faced on the pillows, while the matron gaily chops the cord and whisks your little one off for a good scrub down with some Johnson & Johnson. This is how they used to roll, but these days a lot more is understood about the wonderful benefits of taking a 'hands off' approach at this magical time. However, like everything else, if you really want things done a certain way, you need to put them in your plan and make sure the professionals you are working with know what you want in advance.

More about... Optimal Cord Clamping (OCC)

Sometimes called 'delayed cord clamping', this simply means waiting for at least a minute before cutting the baby's umbilical cord after birth. When the baby is born, at least 30 per cent of their intended blood volume is still in the placenta, but standard practice has been to cut the cord immediately, even before the baby has taken their first breath. Although UK NICE guidelines and international guidelines are now clear that practitioners should wait, unfortunately this does not always happen, which is why it is important to make it clear in your birth plan. A good guide is to wait until the cord is white and has stopped pulsating: some say, 'wait for white'.

Why wait to cut the cord? What's the evidence?

- Your baby will get 30 per cent more of their intended blood volume from the cord and placenta.
- Your baby can gain up to 214g in the first five minutes following birth if the cord is left unclamped.
- Your baby will have increased iron stores and less chance of anaemia if you wait to clamp.

Planning your perfect Hour of Power

Catching your own baby. Traditionally, only 'expert' hands could do the job of 'delivering' a newborn, but many women are now deciding that they want their own hands to be the first to touch their child. It's simple: you reach down, and – with the help of your midwife or by yourself – you bring your baby out and up to your chest for skin-to-skin.

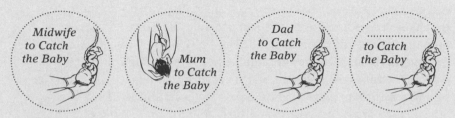

The birth pause. Some women like to leave their baby where they 'land' – if you are on your knees then they will be just there between your legs on the bed – and take a moment to just look at them, before picking them up. We are not talking about a very long time here, maybe less than a minute. But just a little pause to absorb the experience of seeing your baby for the first time. If left undisturbed, some women take this pause instinctively.

The first breath. Babies will take their first breath some time shortly after birth, and it can be beautiful to witness. Some mums like to gently blow on their baby's face to encourage them to take a breath.

Saying hello. Babies are often very alert at birth and if the birth has been calm they are usually calm too. They will often meet your gaze with very wise eyes and you can spend a moment looking at each other's faces. You can gently talk to your baby, telling them that you are their mummy and that you love them – or anything else you think they would like to hear!

Discovering the sex yourself. Many parents find out the sex of their baby during pregnancy, with some having a very public celebration and moment of discovery at so-called 'gender reveal parties' (see page 163). Some wistful and old-fashioned folk (myself included), prefer to wait until the moment of birth, and if you fall into this category it's important to make sure your care providers know not to shout out 'IT'S A BOY!' in *Call the Midwife* style. I can assure you that you don't need any medical training to perform this task yourself, and that it can be really empowering and exciting to take a look and find out if it's 'boy or girl'. And if you can bear the suspense, you can even wait five minutes, half an hour or even longer, to 'fall in love first', before knowing your baby's sex.

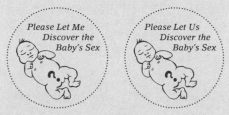

Optimal cord clamping. Over a third of a newborn's blood is still in their placenta and cord at birth. There is no need to cut the cord immediately; it's much better to 'wait for white', until the cord is white and no longer pulsating. There are very few circumstances in which it is not possible to delay cord clamping. This is clear in NICE guidelines, but you may still have to be vocal and insistent to ensure your baby's cord is not cut too soon. (For more see page 103.)

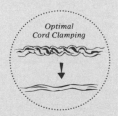

Switching off. It's tempting to get straight on Facebook and give the world a blow-by-blow account of your birth, or at least a pic of your newborn's perfect little nose, but try to wait, at least for a little while, and just 'be here now' as the saying goes. Take in every detail of this moment and enjoy it: social media can wait. However, do take some photos, as you will treasure these in the future.

Skin-to-skin. This means holding your baby, naked, against your bare chest. There are many benefits of skin-to-skin contact, including regulating baby's temperature, reducing stress in both mum and baby, seeding the microbiome, and initiating breastfeeding. (For more info see page 109.)

Delaying wiping or washing. When babies are born, they can have a little blood or amniotic fluid on them, and often they will also have a white, waxy substance known as vernix. This has often been quickly washed or wiped away by health professionals, but there is now evidence to suggest that it's better to leave the vernix alone and delay bathing for a few days. Washing baby down can't be much good for the microbiome (see page 165), and we also know that vernix has moisturising and anti-microbial properties. If you do need to clean away any meconium (baby's first poo), simply use cotton wool and water. Otherwise, leave well alone and revel in the one fragrance that can't be reproduced in a perfume factory: 'Newborn'!

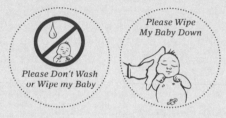

No hats. Hats on newborns is traditional, but some argue this harks back to a time when they were whisked off to the draughty hospital nursery. If a baby is snuggled up under blankets on mum's chest, a hat is surplus to requirements, since mum's body will work miracles to regulate baby's temperature, even raising mum's temperature by as much as a degree if baby is cold. A hat also prevents mum from being able to smell her baby's head, and these olfactory cues are an important aspect of mammalian bonding. If you think that sounds nuts, just sniff your newborn's head: you'll understand immediately.

Keeping it calm. During the Hour of Power, lots of wonderful bonding takes place, and if you want to breastfeed, this is a great time to first offer your baby your breast. Just like birth, bonding and breastfeeding need oxytocin (see page 128), so it's a good idea to try and keep that first hour as calm, dimly lit and free of disruptions as possible, just as your birth room hopefully was. Some women request that non-essential checks like weighing are delayed for at least the first hour, no matter if their baby is born vaginally or by caesarean.

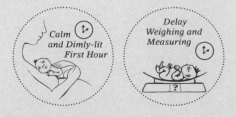

- Your baby will have a higher ratio of red blood cells to the volume of blood (haematocrit), meaning more oxygen to vital organs.
- Your baby will get more stem cells (cord blood is rich in stem cells), which function as building blocks for the immune system and promote long-term health.
- If your baby is premature (see page 238), waiting to clamp decreases the risk of intraventricular haemorrhage, late onset sepsis, necrotising enterocolitis and blood transfusions.
- Waiting to cut the cord may prevent complications in delivering the placenta.

Why cut the cord immediately? What's the evidence?

There is absolutely no evidence whatsoever to support cutting the cord immediately. It's just 'the way things have been done' for a long time, and thankfully, now that the possible detrimental effects are understood, most practitioners are 'waiting for white'.

What if there's an emergency with my baby?

This is often given as a reason to cut the cord early, but in fact NICE guidelines recommend delaying cord clamping regardless of the type of delivery, unless your baby's heart rate is slower than 60 beats per minute and not getting faster. This is extremely rare. If your baby needs to be resuscitated, there is still no reason why this cannot take place with the cord attached. The placenta and cord are still transferring oxygenated blood to your baby, just as they did when the baby was in your womb.

What if I have a caesarean birth?

Waiting to cut the cord is possible at caesarean births, although it is less likely to be common practice. It's a good idea to put it in your Caesarean Birth Plan (page 116) and make sure, like everything else in your plan, that you discuss it in advance with your care providers and get them to sign your birth plan if necessary to say that they have understood your wishes.

Can I still have OCC if I am rhesus negative?

Yes. Your midwife only needs a small sample of blood and this can either be taken from the cord while it is still attached and pulsating, or from the placenta after it has been delivered. It can also be taken from the baby later, as you have a 72-hour window to have the 'anti-D' injection if it is wanted or needed. With new forms of screening being introduced such as NIPT (a blood test in pregnancy to look for chromosomal differences which can also reveal your baby's blood group), testing for blood group at birth may soon become a thing of the past. For more on your choices if you are rhesus negative, see page 254.

> 'Tell the doctor it's against your religion to cut the cord. If you don't have a religion, make one up on the spot. He can't argue with that.'
>
> Ina May Gaskin

What about cord blood banking?

Cord blood banking is big business. While there are some options to donate your baby's cord blood, for example in the NHS, there are many more private companies who charge around £2,000 or more to collect and bank your baby's cord blood, which they often describe as 'a waste product with life-saving potential'. However, you can't do 'optimal clamping' and 'cord blood banking'. So it's worth considering whether you want to donate around a third of your baby's blood volume, by having it banked for their own or anyone else's possible future use. Although we can't predict every scientific advance of the future, it's thought that the chance that your own baby will need their banked cord blood before the age of 20 could be as little as 1 in 20,000. Also, should your child develop leukaemia, it's extremely unlikely that his or her own cord blood will be appropriate for transplant. Essentially, so-called 'cord blood' is actually 'your baby's blood'. Perhaps the health benefits might be highest for your child if this blood goes straight into their body at birth?

In summary

Waiting for the cord to stop pulsating and turn white, and knowing that all your baby's blood has been transferred to them, should not be thought of as an 'option' – it should be standard good practice. However, because professionals have been so used to cutting the cord immediately over the last few decades, it's important that you put it in your plan and make sure that it is not overlooked for any reason.

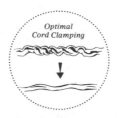

Optimal Cord Clamping

Who will cut the cord?

Dads cutting the cord has become traditional, but there's no reason why you might not want to be the one who makes the final significant move to separate you and your baby. Some women give this rather special privilege to a family member, such as grandma or an older sibling. Others find the thought of it a bit 'ick'; in that case you can always just get the midwife to do it.

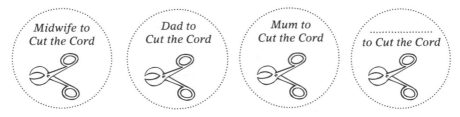

Lotus birth

Some women choose a 'lotus birth': this is when the cord is not cut at all, but left intact to dry up and fall away of its own accord. The process takes around four days, during which time the parents do not welcome any visitors and the placenta, carried along with the baby, is packed in herbs and salt. There are no known health benefits to this practice; rather it is felt to be symbolic of a gentle and natural separation from the mother.

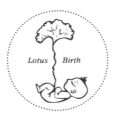

More about... skin-to-skin

Skin-to-skin contact would have been out of the question in the past few decades, when babies were washed, wiped and whisked off to the nursery before mums could say, 'What just happened?'. However, we are thankfully now returning to the practice of babies being placed naked and prone onto mum's chest after birth, which, when you think about it, has probably – along with optimal clamping – been the norm for most of the history of womankind. There are real benefits to skin-to-skin contact with your baby, not least the fact that it just feels like heaven on a stick. Besides the indescribable bliss, other benefits include:

- Thermal regulation: being on your chest will help your baby to maintain the right temperature. Your body will actually warm up if your baby is too cold, and cool down if your baby is too hot. Yes, you really are that clever.
- Your baby's heart rate, breathing rate, blood pressure and blood sugar levels are kept more stable during skin-to-skin.
- Skin-to-skin is brilliant for getting breastfeeding off to a cracking start. Your baby is more likely to latch on (take the nipple and breast in their mouth and begin suckling) and get milk effectively if they are skin-to-skin.
- New research shows that the combination of skin-to-skin contact and breastfeeding – which the researchers have named 'pronurturance' – can significantly reduce the possibility of post-birth haemorrhage.
- Skin-to-skin is an important part of the process of 'seeding the microbiome' (see page 165). We know that babies placed in an incubator are often colonised by different bacteria to those of their mother.
- If you are unwell at or after the birth, skin-to-skin may still be possible. Even after a caesarean under general anaesthetic (see page 214), you might still be able to have your baby placed on your chest, albeit not immediately. If you are uncomfortable or unable to do skin-to-skin, your partner or a close relative can take your place; it will be a positive and bonding experience for them too.
- Skin-to-skin is highly beneficial in the first hour of life, but it doesn't have to end there – you can carry on having skin-to-skin as much as you like and as often as you like for the first days and weeks of your baby's life. The benefits continue.

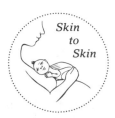

 Please note: skin-to-skin means what it says on the tin. No blankets wrapped around baby, just their naked skin, on your naked skin. Skin-to-skin!

What about the third stage?

Some women choose to have 'active management' – an injection of syntometrine or syntocinon to encourage the placenta to come out. A Cochrane review of both drugs has found that syntometrine is more effective than syntocinon in reducing blood loss during the delivery of the placenta, but that it has more side-effects, so you may wish to discuss this further with your midwife and find out which you are more likely to be given and if you would prefer to choose one over the other. Alternatively, you can choose to have a natural or 'physiological' third stage.

Physiological third stage

If you've had a drug-free labour you might be inclined to continue this trend by declining the injection, which is administered into your thigh shortly after the birth. Your body is well designed to expel the placenta, and in most cases this is what happens, usually between 10 minutes and an hour after the birth. During this time you can hold your baby, and they can remain attached to their umbilical cord, or, if it has stopped pulsating, the cord can be clamped and cut if you wish. Breastfeeding during this time can also help your uterus to contract and expel the placenta.

Active management and delayed active management

For many years, the injection of syntometrine or syntocinon – given because there is some evidence that getting the placenta out in this way reduces the risk of haemorrhage – was given immediately after birth or even during the delivery. Some have raised concerns that this makes immediate cord clamping necessary, in case any of the injected drug transfers to the baby. However, the NICE guidelines still recommend giving the injection at birth, in spite of their guidance to delay cord clamping by one to five minutes, as they say the amount of syntometrine that passes to the baby is not enough to cause concern. Others disagree; in New Zealand guidelines say that the injection should be given after delayed clamping has taken place. This is called 'delayed active management'. It is up to you whether you choose a physiological third stage (no injection), active management (immediate injection) or waiting until after the cord is cut to have the injection (delayed active management).

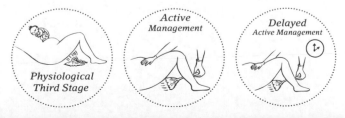

Physiological Third Stage   *Active Management*   *Delayed Active Management*

Do you want to keep your placenta?

If your answer to this question is an immediate 'Ew, nope!', then skip this bit. While some of us would rather lick the pub floor than even so much as look at a placenta, others find it a fascinating and beautiful part of the birth process. Here are a few ideas of what you could do with your placenta if you don't want it whisked away immediately.

Look at it. Some call the placenta the 'Tree of Life', and if you have a look at your baby's placenta, you will see why. It's got a rather amazing structure, with the 'trunk' coming up from the umbilical cord, and lots of tiny 'branches' fanning out from this. Each one is different and unique and you might like to see what yours looks like out of sheer curiosity.

Eat it. Yes, people do this, and many swear by it, saying that consuming the organ, either raw or in capsules, gave them wonderful postnatal energy or even staved off post-natal depression. Unfortunately, there isn't any official evidence to support these claims, but there are certainly a lot of women (and of course some celebrities) who say it has benefited them. If you want to eat yours, some women put a thin sliver into a fruit smoothie (look online for guidelines and recipes), or for around £150 you can pay a professional to dry it, crush it into powder, and deliver it in capsule form. For the latter, visit IPEN (see resources).

Bury it. Many other cultures honour the significance of the placenta; the Navajo and the Maori, for example, give it a ritual burial, believing it binds the child to its ancestral land and people. Some other cultures see the placenta as a lost twin, or the place where a child's guardian spirit resides. If you feel that the placenta has some significance for you, you may like to bury it, perhaps under a special tree that can grow as your child grows. You may have to wait a year if you are planting a new tree though, as the high iron levels in the placenta can kill off new plants.

 In the Maori language, the words for 'placenta' and 'land' are the same: whenua.

Make placenta prints. You or your midwives or helpers can lie the placenta on acid-free paper to make a print. The result looks like a 'leaf print', or a very stylised tree. Some women later add to the print with coloured paints or other decorations to make a very unique piece of art.

Cord art. This involves placing the cord into a shape, often a heart, and either photographing it (sometimes when baby and placenta are still attached), or drying it (sometimes done by the person who encapsulates it) as a keepsake.

If you do want to keep your placenta, don't forget you'll need a container for it. If you are encapsulating it your specialist will probably provide you with a kit or advice. If you want to bury it or just wait a while before you decide what to do with it, your best bet is to stick it in your freezer. Just make sure you don't mistake it for a beef madras in your post-partum haze and optimistically stick it on defrost in the microwave while the rice is cooking.

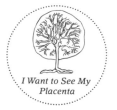
I Want to See My Placenta

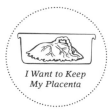
I Want to Keep My Placenta

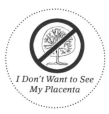
I Don't Want to See My Placenta

How do you plan to feed your baby?

It's worth stating on your birth plan your intention to either breastfeed or formula feed. This might be especially helpful if your baby is premature or poorly or you are separated for any reason. Breastfeeding expert Emma Pickett (see page 278) also recommends you write a Breastfeeding Plan to accompany your VBP, with reminders about skin-to-skin, how and when you want the first feed to happen, and useful resources for support.

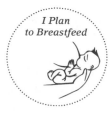
I Plan to Breastfeed

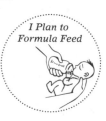
I Plan to Formula Feed

Vitamin K: yay or nay?

Vitamin K is offered to all newborns in the UK, either in the form of an injection or as oral drops. This is because research has shown that some newborns have low levels of vitamin K, which plays a role in blood clotting. Low vitamin K levels can thus cause a condition known as Haemorrhagic Disease of the Newborn (HDN), also known as Vitamin K Deficiency Bleeding (VKDB).

VKDB is a rare but unpredictable occurrence in which a baby will start to bleed – from various sites including the skin, brain, abdomen, nose or mouth – in the first few days or weeks of life.

How likely this bleeding is to have severe consequences depends on how old the baby is when it occurs, and how easy the bleed is to notice – bleeding in the brain, for example, can be hard to detect in small babies before damage has already occurred.

It's frustrating, of course, that we don't currently have any way of predicting which babies will develop VKDB and which will be fine. This means that we are giving an injection of vitamin K to thousands of babies who don't really need it. But as it stands, this has been deemed the best way to prevent the worst-case scenario of brain damage or death in a small minority.

In spite of this, there are widespread misconceptions about vitamin K, and many parents in both the UK and the USA are declining the vitamin K injection. This is an unfortunate side-effect, perhaps, of the drive towards less intervention in birth. Of course, I fully support this drive, but it's also important not to take a polarised approach and risk throwing the baby out with the bath water. Some interventions and advances in medical science can be vital and life-saving, and it seems like vitamin K could be one such intervention.

A quick internet search about vitamin K will lead you to sites which give you some of the following information, which might worry you if you are researching your choices:

- The vitamin K injection is linked to childhood cancer
- The injection is unnatural and full of toxins that will harm your baby
- Delayed cord clamping negates the need for the injection
- You don't need the injection if you had a gentle or natural birth
- There must be a reason for the deficiency in newborns; 'mother nature would not get it wrong'.

However, Rebecca Dekker, Professor of Nursing and author of the website Evidence Based Birth, points out that most of these articles are written by people who have no healthcare or research background and that there is actually no evidence for any of these claims. Dekker has thoroughly reviewed all the available evidence about vitamin K. Her findings include:

- There is no evidence of a link between the vitamin K shot and childhood cancer
- Delayed cord clamping has not been shown in research to raise vitamin K levels
- There is no evidence that supplementing the maternal diet with vitamin K during pregnancy or breastfeeding can raise levels in the baby
- There is no evidence to support the claim that babies who have had a traumatic birth are more at risk of VKDB
- A 'preservative free' version of the injection can be requested and this contains plant-based products, salt, vinegar and propylene glycol (recognised as safe by the FDA for use in food products)
- Exclusively formula-fed babies have virtually zero risk of VKDB. This is because, in contrast to breastmilk, formula contains relatively high levels of vitamin K
- Injected vitamin K is more effective than oral drops, especially in preventing 'late VKDB', which can occur in weeks 2 to 12 of life.

If you choose to give vitamin K, it will be given as an injection at birth, or via oral drops on day 1, day 5 to 7, and for breastfed babies a final dose at 28 days. An alternative called Neokay – vitamin K in coconut oil – can be given as a weekly oral dose for 12 weeks. Even formula-fed babies will be offered vitamin K, as VKDB can occur in the first 24 hours of life and the injection at birth prevents this. If you decline, you may like to be especially aware of the signs of VKDB, which include blood oozing from the cord stump, prolonged bleeding after the heel-prick test, a nose bleed or unexplained bruising. If you have any concerns, see your doctor or midwife immediately, regardless of whether or not you have chosen vitamin K.

As always, whether or not you choose the vitamin K injection, the oral drops, or you decline both, is entirely up to you. It's important to stress that VKDB is very rare. For example, between 4 and 10 babies in 100,000 will develop VKDB after the first week of life. That's not a very significant number – unless your baby happens to be one of them. So it's also important to consider that no babies at all who have the injection will go on to develop VKDB.

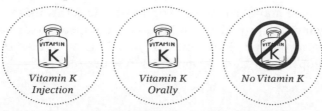

Vitamin K Injection   Vitamin K Orally   No Vitamin K

Making a caesarean plan: the 'Best Possible Caesarean' or BPC

Whether you know in advance that you are having a caesarean birth, or whether you think you're going to give birth in a tent in your garden (yes, it's been done), you need to make a plan for your 'Best Possible Caesarean' (BPC). This doesn't mean you are going to have a caesarean – you might not! Nor does it mean you are going to love your caesarean – although many women do, and you might be one of them. But thinking about a BPC means that you are able to reclaim the experience of giving birth by caesarean and feel actively involved in it. This will really help you as you think about it afterwards.

Many of the icons and choices that you've already read about in this chapter can be transferred to your BPC plan. You may also like to consider some or all of the elements of a 'gentle' or 'woman-centred caesarean' (for all the info you need, see page 208). If so, the extra icons you may find helpful are:

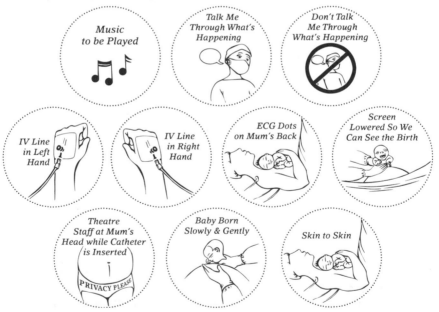

So your BPC plan might look something like the sample on the following two pages.

If you want a gentle caesarean you do need to remember this is unlikely to be 'standard', so you will need to talk through your plan with your care providers, and if necessary speak to different consultants in your hospital or even, if your BPC is planned in advance, shop around at different units in your area.

Charlie & Sam: Best Possible Caesarean Plan
(St Mary's Hospital, Treestone)

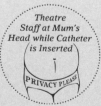
Caesarean Birth

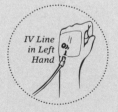
Theatre Birth

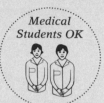
Medical Students OK

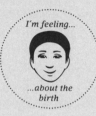
I'm feeling... ...about the birth

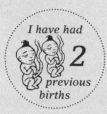
I have had 2 previous births

Survivor of Abuse

Music to be Played

Quiet Please No Chatting

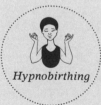
Hypnobirthing

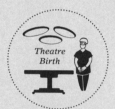
IV Line in Left Hand

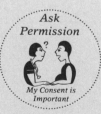
Ask Permission My Consent is Important

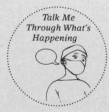
Talk Me Through What's Happening

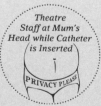
Theatre Staff at Mum's Head while Catheter is Inserted PRIVACY PLEASE

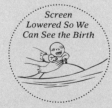
Screen Lowered So We Can See the Birth

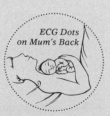
ECG Dots on Mum's Back

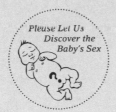

Please Let Us Discover the Baby's Sex

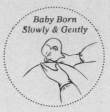

Baby Born Slowly & Gently

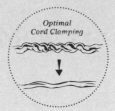

Optimal Cord Clamping

Please Don't Wash or Wipe my Baby

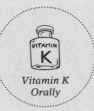

Vitamin K Orally

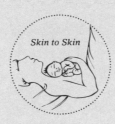

Skin to Skin

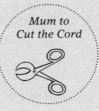

Mum to Cut the Cord

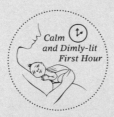

Calm and Dimly-lit First Hour

Delay Weighing and Measuring

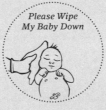

Please Wipe My Baby Down

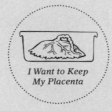

I Want to Keep My Placenta

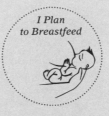

I Plan to Breastfeed

Making plans B, C & D: when birth doesn't go to plan

By now you should have thought about all aspects of your birth choices, and you probably have a fairly clear idea of your Plan A. But of course, birth may not go exactly the way you want. Really good birth preparation is a two-pronged attack: you need to learn as much as you can about how you can maximise your chances of birth going exactly as you want, and you need to think about what it might be like if it doesn't. This is where Plan B comes in. And C. And D.

Think in advance of as many scenarios as you can and what you would like to happen. For example, if you are planning a home birth, but find you have to transfer to hospital, it's really important that you have considered in advance what you want from a hospital birth experience, what you will and will not consent to, and how you can make it the best birth it can be.

Remember too that if you are asked to deviate from the original plan, it's unusual for the emergency to be so serious that you have to make an immediate decision. You should take time, perhaps along with your partner, to consider the course of action that feels right for you. When doing so, many people find the BRAIN acronym really helpful.

Making decisions in labour with BRAIN

Ask yourself...

B – What are the Benefits?
Ask your healthcare professional what the benefits are of the intervention that is being offered, and consider what you feel the benefits will be to you personally. For example, might breaking your waters get your labour moving and would this be a positive thing for you?

R – What are the Risks?
Find out what the risks are that come with this procedure. Ask for the clear facts and the evidence upon which they are based.

A – What are the Alternatives?
Are there other options or courses of action that you could take? Ask what they are and apply your BRAIN to them too!

I – What does your Intuition tell you?
Listen to your instincts and tune into your body and your baby.
Trust that, deep down, you know the best course of action for
you and your baby.

N – What happens if we do Nothing?
Ask your healthcare professional what will happen if you just
wait and see what happens, for 10 minutes, half an hour, or
more. You might appreciate this time to take the pressure off,
breathe, and reflect.

Bringing a new life into the world involves a strange mix of fully
and consciously preparing and then completely surrendering to the
process of birth. However, it's really important to remember that even
if birth deviates a long, long way from your hopes, there should still be
elements from your original plan, for example optimal clamping, that
you can retain in almost any circumstance.

Use my HEART acronym to remind yourself and your partner of a
few vital elements when birth doesn't go the way you had hoped.

Birthing from your HEART

Ask yourself…

H – How can I keep the important Hormones flowing?
Oxytocin – known as the 'love hormone' – helps with birthing,
bonding and breastfeeding. The hormone of fight, flight and
panic – adrenaline – inhibits its release. It might help to dim
the lights or ask for some quiet time alone together without
interruptions – even for 10 minutes – so you can get back in
a relaxation 'zone' and kick-start your mammalian instincts.
If there simply isn't time for this, try to focus on love – love
for your partner and love for your baby – and aim to banish
adrenaline and welcome back oxytocin. Birthing with love, even
in theatre, can mean better bonding and breastfeeding, and
more positive memories after the event.

E – What Elements of my birth plan can I retain?
Just because birth is not going the way you wished, doesn't mean
you have to completely abandon every single one of your hopes.
If you wanted certain music playing, for example, might this still

be possible? Or can it be played soon after the birth instead? Or if you wanted skin-to-skin, can this still be arranged? If not, ask why not. If something is important to you, try to keep it in your plans.

A – Baby in Arms as soon as possible.

No matter how you birth, try to make sure your baby comes to you as soon as possible afterwards. Even if medical complications mean that this is not immediate, try to make sure that both you and your partner get to experience this unique time of meeting your baby. Try to get someone to take a photo, as many mums say that they really treasure these pictures at a later date. Make this your priority. Everything else can wait.

R – Find your Resilience

When the going gets tough… call on a mum. Mums have strength and courage by the bucket load, and many of them first contact this warrior side of themselves as they struggle to bring their babies into the world. You may not feel strong as your birth plans fly out of the window, but you are. You may not feel strong in the days and weeks after you've given birth, especially if you've had a difficult or traumatic experience, but you are. You might need help and support to recover – and it takes strength to ask for this. But recover you will, and in that process, remember the strength that brought your baby into the world, and draw on it as you move forwards into the many and various challenges of motherhood.

T – Allow yourself Time.

Birth is a big deal. Women remember minute details from their birth for the rest of their lives. Don't be discouraged from taking what happened to you in your birth experience seriously. If you lost track of Plan A or even Plan B, you have a right to feel sad, disappointed, or traumatised. You have a right to grieve this loss. It doesn't mean that you don't love or appreciate your healthy baby. Take your time. You matter too.

Whether or not you decide to make a VBP, you might like to write a longer birth plan with more detailed information about you and your preferences. These samples will give you a better idea of how you might do this, but of course your birth plan is personal and will ultimately be unique to you and your choices.

Sample Birth Plan I

Emily and Rob's plan for a home birth

Overview – our aim is to have a natural birth, at home, with as little intervention as possible. We would like the event itself to be an enjoyable and life-enhancing experience, rather than something to be feared or got through as quickly as possible.

However – we remain realistic about the possibility that it is unlikely that everything will go as planned, and are willing to listen to the advice of professionals and seek medical attention should this be necessary.

General

Induction – we would prefer induction to be used as a last resort, and would prefer to be left to go into spontaneous labour, so long as all is well with Emily and the baby.

Pain Relief – we would like to avoid the use of medication unless the labour is very long or difficult. We would like to have gas and air available for a home birth. Whether at home or in hospital, Emily would prefer not to be offered pain relief during labour, but would rather ask for herself should she wish to try it. Emily does not wish to have an epidural.

Other Interventions – we would prefer any other interventions, such as drugs to augment labour, forceps, ventouse, caesarean etc, not to be used, except as an absolute last resort.

Lighting – whether at home or in hospital, please leave the lighting as dim as possible, including after the birth.

Atmosphere – we would prefer to create our own atmosphere in the birth room, particularly if we are in hospital. This may include music, pictures or photos on the wall, our own pillows, birth ball etc.

Support – Emily would like Rob to be her main support during labour, and to give birth in a quiet and calm atmosphere in which they are able to focus together on the task in hand.

Transfer to Hospital – should this be necessary Emily would like Rob to remain with her at all times. In the ambulance please do not strap Emily on her back; she would prefer to be on her side.

Student Doctors/Midwives – if in hospital we do not wish to be observed by students or any other people, other than the necessary minimum.

First Stage

Cervical Examinations – only at our request please.

Continuous Electronic Foetal Monitoring – no thanks. Any necessary monitoring to be done with Sonicaid or ear trumpet please.

Alternative Remedies – we wish to use massage, aromatherapy, homeopathy and herbal remedies during the labour.

Freedom of Movement – Emily wishes to have an active birth and be free to move around at will, choosing positions herself that she finds helpful.

Food and Drink – Emily wishes to continue to eat and drink as and when she wishes during labour.

Waters – please do not break Emily's waters artificially, unless, as with all other interventions, this is felt to be absolutely necessary. If so please discuss with us first.

Talking – we would like the room to be quiet and calm in atmosphere. Please do not talk, in particular during contractions. If there are practical matters to discuss, e.g. between midwives, please do this out of the room.

Second Stage

Pushing – In the second stage, Emily would like to push in her own way and in her own time, rather than being directed, unless she requests otherwise. After transition, please allow Emily to rest a while if she has no pushing urge.

Episiotomy – we would prefer not to have this procedure. Should Emily have a 1st degree tear she would prefer to be left to heal naturally.

Time – unless there are evidence-based concerns about the welfare of the baby or Emily, or both, she does not wish 'time' to be a factor in any decision-making regarding interventions or transfers to hospital. She would prefer it if those attending her did not talk to her or each other about time.

The Birth

Catching the Baby – we wish Rob to be the person to do this if possible.

Boy or Girl – we would like to find out the baby's sex ourselves, rather than being told.

Cutting the Cord – we would like Rob to cut the cord or to cut the cord together. We wish to wait until the cord has stopped pulsating and changed colour before it is clamped or cut.

Third Stage

Third Stage – we would prefer to have a physiological third stage and deliver the placenta without a syntometrine injection unless we are given good reason why this is absolutely necessary.

Placenta – if at home we would like to put this in a bag in the deep freeze so that we can bury it somewhere special. If in hospital we would like to take it home with us.

First Hour – we would like the baby to be placed immediately on Emily's tummy/breast for skin-to-skin contact. We would like the baby to remain unclothed. We would like any weighing, measuring etc to be delayed for at least an hour so that all three of us have time to bond. We consider this to be a really important time for everyone.

Afterwards

First Day/Night(s) – should we be in hospital we would like the baby to remain with Emily and/or Rob at all times.

Feeding – we wish to breastfeed and hope that this can begin naturally soon after the birth. However, if necessary we would like help and support with this.

Vitamin K – we wish to administer oral drops rather than the baby have an injection.

Sample Birth Plan II

This birth plan was used by Frederique and Aaron, who planned a gentle or woman-centred elective caesarean birth for their fourth baby.

Aaron and I are looking forward to sharing our first caesarean birth experience with you.

This plan outlines some of our preferences for birth and we hope that you'll help us move towards our goals as much as possible to make the birth of our baby a sacred experience.

We would like to be informed at all times of any procedures or medications to be allowed the chance to give our informed consent.

Thank you!

Companion during Labour – Aaron (husband)
We would like my husband to stay throughout.

Prior to Surgery

Preparing a Vaginal Swab – We strongly believe in 'seeding and feeding our baby's microbiome'.
We would like to prepare a vaginal swab to be used immediately onto our baby after delivery.

During Surgery

Medications – Please ensure that all medications are suitable for breastfeeding

I would like a regional anaesthetic

I would like non-drowsy medications

No sedatives after the birth

Screen – I wish to have no screen throughout the procedure

Slower Procedure or 'Natural' C-section – If possible, could you 'walk' Baby slowly out of my womb to allow for a slower birth and help the fluids out of the lungs.

If allowed and obviously discussed and planned prior to the surgery, I would be keen to participate in a 'Maternal Assisted Caesarean' and be able to deliver my baby myself or at least be able to place my hands on Baby's head as s/he is lifted out.

Please allow for skin-to-skin contact immediately after delivery and evaluate Baby on my chest. (If this is not possible – then father would like skin-to-skin contact)

Delayed Cord Clamping – If possible allow the cord to continue pulsing after the birth so Baby may start breathing on her/his own while still attached to the placenta

Sex of Baby – We would like to discover the sex of our baby ourselves

Vaginal Swab – We would like Baby to be swabbed as soon as possible after delivery

Stitches – I would prefer dissolvable stitches

Placenta – We wish to keep my placenta and will provide a container to place it in

After Surgery

Vitamin K – We wish our baby to be given oral vitamin K

Feeding my Baby – I would like to breastfeed my baby and would appreciate all the support and encouragement you can give me to exclusively breastfeed

OK, I've made an Uber Birth Plan. What do I do with it now?

Now that you've got this awesome document that has taken you so much time and thought, your next task is to make sure it's read. This might, at times, make you feel like J. K. Rowling trying to find a publisher for a little-known book about a wizard, but remember: she got there in the end.

First of all, make sure that anyone who is going to be at your birth reads your plan and talks it over with you in detail. Your partner, mum, and doula may want to have input, but remember, birth is your party, and while you will of course want to listen to their views, you don't have to change your plans to suit other people, and the buck stops with you. It's vital that those attending your birth are up to speed and on board with your wishes, as when labour intensifies, they may be more able to advocate for your wishes than you are.

Secondly, you need to make sure your midwives and care providers have read your plan. It's worth discussing every element with them, giving particular focus to any areas that might deviate from the 'standard'. For example, if you don't want to have routine VEs in labour, or if you want a gentle caesarean (see page 208), you can't – unfortunately – just turn up on the day and expect this to happen. It's much better to get all your care providers on board with your wishes before the birth. Meet with senior midwives or others involved in decisions about your care, and ask them to record the discussions and the decisions that you have made, and sign your birth plan. These discussions should be helpful to both parties: your care providers can demonstrate that they have fulfilled their obligation to have a balanced and individualised discussion with you about your personal circumstances and risk factors, and you can demonstrate that you have understood the information given to you and that your wishes have been documented. Your birth plan will not have legal status, but it is still evidence that your views and preferences have been discussed and noted.

❧ Chapter 7 ☙

Pregnant Pause

This is the tea and biscuits part of the book. You've done the hard stuff, challenging your age-old assumptions, making a birth plan, stressing about vitamin K, and arguing about epidurals with the man in the pub. That bit was tough. Time to grab a blanket and relax.

Dunk your digestives and find out more about everything from the fabulous love hormone oxytocin to the wonders of water birth; from the magic of knowing your midwife to the best positions for labour for both you and your baby; from the power of your mind over your body, to the exciting new science of the human microbiome.

From where to find the best available research and evidence, to what to pack in your birth bag, there's vital information in this part of the book that could make all the difference to your experience of pregnancy or the kind of birth you end up having. Let your baby (and your biscuits) slowly expand your body, as this chapter gently expands your mind to match.

The vital role of oxytocin

If you're packing your hospital bag, or getting the room all ready for your home birth, it's a safe bet that you've forgotten one vital item. You can't give birth without it, and you have to provide your own. It's free, the supply is unlimited, but ignore it at your birth peril. No friends, it's not inco sheets or paper pants, it's the wonder hormone, oxytocin.

Put simply, even if you forget everything else, you need to make sure that oxytocin is at your birth in extremely large quantities.

Oxytocin – sometimes known as the 'love hormone' – is produced by your body when you feel safe, happy, warm, cosy and emotionally liberated. You produce it when you are falling head over heels in love. You produce it when you are having really good sex. You produce it when you are breastfeeding, and one day, although this might be hard to visualise right now, you will produce it when you tiptoe into your child's bedroom and see how beautiful they look when they're sleeping.

And guess what, oxytocin is the most important hormone in the birth process.

It's the driving force behind every labour contraction, and works so well to get things moving along that women are often given a synthetic version of it in a drip (Syntocinon or pitocin) to speed their labour up or just to get it going in the first place.

The good news is that you can make your own abundant supply; the bad news is that oxytocin is also known as the 'shy hormone'. Essentially, if you think about the circumstances under which you would have the best sex of your life, versus the circumstances where you would, quite frankly, rather die than have an orgasm, you are already half way to a degree in Oxytocin Studies. Before you get distracted, let's get you that certificate...

Oxytocin likes: darkness, safety, quiet, warmth, privacy, love. It likes massage, people who whisper, 'You're beautiful', tea-lights, and compilation playlists.

Oxytocin does not like: interruptions, bright lights, strangers, cold, fear, unfamiliarity. It does not like people chit-chatting while it is trying to get in the zone, or TVs on in the background, or rough poky fingers.

Oxytocin is the reason home birth makes a lot of sense. Most of us would rather get jiggy on our own sofa than in a stark delivery room observed by a woman called Barbara we'd only just met (although there's no accounting for taste). For the same reasons, our chances of producing the labour hormone oxytocin may well be higher at home: in hospital, we may 'fail to progress'. In fact, this often happens: women who feel like they are moving towards the 'cracking on phase' at home dash to the hospital in a state of panic, only to find that all signs of their labour seem to have disappeared. They get sent home, and everything slowly gets going again. As they say in America, you do the math.

But this doesn't mean to say that home birth is the only way. Armed with our knowledge of oxytocin, we can seriously up our chances of a positive hospital birth, and dads and partners can really help with this. Often the partner who is not doing the work of labour can feel like a spare part in the delivery room, but if you make them read this bit of the book, they can have a new sense of purpose as they rise to the challenge of being… drum roll… Guardians of Oxytocin!

Guardians of Oxytocin: a nuts and bolts guide for dads and partners

- Women need oxytocin to labour effectively.
- Oxytocin is a 'shy hormone'; we produce it most when we feel safe, when it's calm, quiet and dark.
- Think of the labour room as a cave, with you at the door (loincloth optional) keeping the predators at bay. Guard her space. Guard her oxytocin.
- Make sure that those people who do come in do so quietly, calmly, and don't chitchat. Encourage hushed tones. Make the room dark if you can.
- Adrenaline – the hormone of fear, fight, and flight – is the enemy of oxytocin: it blocks its production. So think about how you can ward off adrenaline and keep it at bay (shining armour optional).
- Make your partner feel beautiful and loved. Kiss, massage and caress her if this is what she wants. Hold her in the warmth of your love from a distance if she needs this instead. Follow her lead, just as you (hopefully) do in the bedroom.
- Learn about the mammal brain and the neocortex (see page 143). Do all of the above and more to help your partner stay in the 'zone' of labour and not be drawn back into her 'thinking' mind. Don't ask her questions or chat to her. Be quiet and let her be.
- Remember that your partner may look very different in labour to the way you usually see her. Her internal experience will be very different to how she looks from the outside. She may feel very powerful, for example, but look out of control. Make a pact that if she needs rescuing, she will ask. Otherwise, assume she doesn't.

If you don't have your baby's dad or a birth partner to help guard your oxytocin, consider hiring a doula (see page 153), or thinking about ways that you can promote the production of this hormone yourself. For example:

- Have photos of people or places you love, or happy times in your life, near you in your birth space.
- During pregnancy, take time out each day to breathe and visualise happy and loving times and places. Call on these visualisations in labour.
- Connect with your baby, if this feels right to you, and focus on your love for them. Imagine this love growing every day once they have been born. Talk to them in your mind as you go through the journey of labour together. They are your ultimate birth partner!
- Try to make your birth space, wherever that may be, as dimly lit, cosy and safe feeling as you can.
- Build a nest or even 'hide' in your birth place. Use sheets or blankets, ear plugs, or an eye mask, to block out light and audio/visual stimulation.
- Stimulate your nipples or your clitoris during labour, as this will raise your oxytocin levels. This is particularly effective if labour stalls and you want to get things moving.

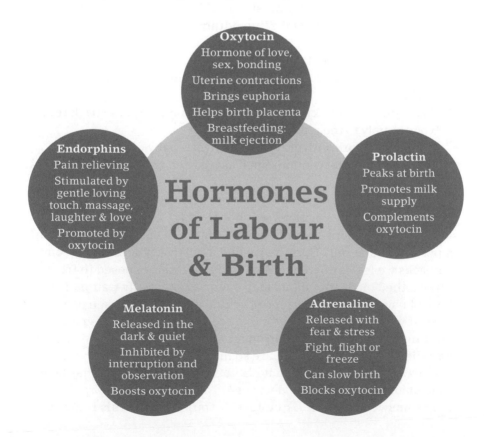

Oxytocin
Hormone of love, sex, bonding
Uterine contractions
Brings euphoria
Helps birth placenta
Breastfeeding: milk ejection

Endorphins
Pain relieving
Stimulated by gentle loving touch. massage, laughter & love
Promoted by oxytocin

Hormones of Labour & Birth

Prolactin
Peaks at birth
Promotes milk supply
Complements oxytocin

Melatonin
Released in the dark & quiet
Inhibited by interruption and observation
Boosts oxytocin

Adrenaline
Released with fear & stress
Fight, flight or freeze
Can slow birth
Blocks oxytocin

Getting off your back

Picture a woman in labour and what do you see? For most of us, the vision is instant: a bed, and a woman on her back. In fact, the figures show that this vision represents reality: one survey suggests around 85 per cent of UK women give birth on a bed. What's more, over half of women deliver babies lying on their backs, and 35 per cent of women are not only on their backs, but have their feet in stirrups too. In America the figures are even higher, with over 90 per cent of women in back-lying positions during the pushing stage and birth.

This seems rather strange. Some 30 years ago or more campaigners were already calling for birthing women to get off their backs. Janet Balaskas pioneered the Active Birth Movement in the early 1980s, and in 1982 thousands of women, led by another birth activist, Sheila Kitzinger, marched on London to defend a woman's right to birth in any position she chose.

And never mind the activists – there's actually plenty of solid evidence that moving freely in labour and choosing your own position for delivery bring real benefits, including:

- Shorter, less painful labour
- Pelvic opening is wider and baby more able to manoeuvre round mother's bones
- Baby gets a better oxygen supply, because lying on the back reduces blood supply to the placenta
- Mother can work with gravity to bring the baby down
- Less need for interventions such as assisted delivery and caesarean

And the benefits of giving birth more actively don't stop at the physical. The bodily positions we choose affect how we feel in all sorts of life situations – ever been told that trick of standing up for an important phone call? Upright, we feel assertive, whereas lying on our backs we feel vulnerable. Having our genitals exposed in front of fully-clothed birth attendants may even be potentially traumatic for those of us who have experienced sexual abuse or rape (see page 92).

So, if we get off the bed, we can have a faster labour, less pain, fewer interventions and feel stronger and more empowered – what's not to like? And why the heck are so many of us still giving birth like this when the message that it's not going to help us out has been shouted loud and strong for decades?

The answer, of course, is 'culture'. In other words, 'this is how we do things round here', or 'monkey see, monkey do'. We actually expect to give birth in this way as this is the most usual image we've seen of birth on TV. Perhaps, too, caregivers might find it more convenient to keep things as they are – after all, this is how women ended up on their backs in the first place, as this position gives attendants the best possible view of proceedings. And with the bed as the central object in almost every hospital birth room, who can blame us if we dutifully get on it?

Right now, the idea of giving birth on a bed is so engrained that most of us just can't imagine anything else. When I planned my first birth, I told a friend, a mother already, of my plans to build a big 'nest' of cushions and blankets on the floor. She frowned: 'But how will they examine you if they have bad backs?' she asked, which got me worried, until another friend, also a mother, but a rather subversive midwife too, assured me that they'd be OK. 'They don't spend the whole labour with their fingers stuck in you, Milli.'

Joking aside, it is difficult to break with convention, and to wrap our heads around the idea that it doesn't matter how our carers feel about our birth choices – we are the ones doing the amazing work of having a baby and we don't need to protect their backs or their feelings.

Don't be afraid to challenge the norm, by turning up for your hospital birth with a yoga mat, birth ball, or – as I once did – a big bag of cushions for your floor nest.

If the idea of this makes you feel uncomfortable, you might first have to challenge your own perceptions and expectations of birth, and dismiss any worries you might have about your choices being inconvenient to others. In other words, as the birth activists of the 1980s would have put it: don't take it lying down.

Your baby's position

If you turn to page 135, you'll see a few suggested positions for an active labour, that you can find either by yourself or with the support of your partner. But what about the position of your baby? If your baby is 'breech' (see page 256) – head at the top rather than near the exit – then you'll find out quite quickly how a bottom-first baby can be a total bummer. But if they are the opposite – 'head down' – then this is OK, right?

Midwife Jean Sutton and antenatal teacher Pauline Scott think it's a bit more complex. In the mid-1990s they published a book explaining that there are actions a mum-to-be can take in pregnancy to ensure that her baby is in the best possible position for labour. They called this Optimal Foetal Positioning, or OFP.

What is the best position for the baby to be in for birth?

Sutton and Scott say that the easiest births happen when the baby is LOA. This stands for Left Occiput Anterior, and basically means head down, facing your back, with their back on the left side to the front of your tummy. Occasionally they may be ROA (Right Occiput Anterior), but this is not quite as ideal, due to the way that the baby has to rotate out of your pelvis.

The theory is that with our more sedentary lifestyles, we lean back more, sitting in car seats, or flopping around on sofas, and we therefore create a 'hammock' in our uterus that encourages the baby to take up an OP (Occiput Posterior) position – with their back to our back. Manual work like scrubbing floors and harvesting, that would have encouraged the baby to take the OA position, is not the way most modern women spend their time. Hashtag TFFT!

Sutton and Scott suggest paying attention to your posture during your pregnancy, avoiding positions where you are lying back or putting your feet up, and making time for activities like yoga, swimming with your belly down in the water, being on all fours and leaning on a chair or birth ball while watching TV, using a wedge to keep your pelvis tilted forwards while driving, and sleeping on your side, all of which can help your baby get into the optimal position for birth. A poorly positioned baby may make birth longer, or more painful, or cause issues like a stop-start first stage or a lack of progress when you are 'pushing'.

Oh no! OP!

So, you can use OFP techniques in pregnancy to encourage your baby to take up the LOA position, but – here's the bad news – many babies who have obediently spent the last weeks of pregnancy 'back to front' can suddenly turn 'back to back', or OP, during labour. In fact, research has found that about two-thirds of babies who are born OP, were OA at the start of labour. Little blighters. And so a lifetime of disobedience begins.

If your baby is OP at the start of labour, or even turns this way during labour, there are still things that you can do to help yourself take control of the situation.

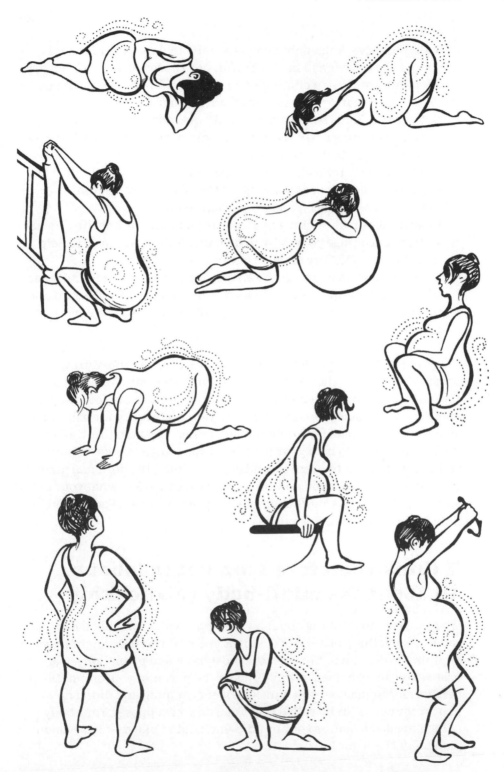

Positions in labour (illustrations by Kate Evans)

- Think positive. You might be persistently told that your labour is going to be harder and more painful, but allow yourself to keep an open mind and use techniques from the mind-body section below to prevent negative expectations from becoming a reality.
- Don't panic. Some babies are born OP and others turn during labour. Like breech, OP could be thought of as 'another variation of normal', rather than 'a problem'.
- In early labour, try techniques to open the pelvis and help the baby wiggle through, such as walking up stairs sideways, marching on the spot, or stepping on and off a small stool.
- In later labour, try rocking in all-fours positions, or kneeling on one knee, to encourage your baby to take up an OA position or to help them be born OP. Stay off your back.
- Your doula or midwife may be able to suggest other ideas and some will use a technique called 'Rebozo', which comes from Mexico and involves supporting you in helpful positions using a large piece of fabric.

There are other awkward positions your baby can get into during pregnancy or birth, such as transverse (lying sideways) or asynclitic (head tilted). OFP techniques are not guaranteed to work, but they will allow you to become more connected to your body and your baby, and to take an active role in your labour, encouraging you to think about the best positions to help your baby be born, and giving you some techniques to try if they are in a difficult position. In short, learning more about how what you do with your body, can affect what your baby will do with theirs, is another great string to your bow. (For helpful links to more info, see Resources.)

'I think therefore I am not in labour': all about the mind-body relationship

We're so used to thinking about birth in physical terms that it can come as something of a shock to consider that our minds might have anything to do with it. But even the most basic and primal physical processes can be helped or hindered by the power of your mind. Don't believe me? Remember that time you went camping and didn't do a poo for four days? Who called that shot, do you suppose? Your body (which needed to go), or your mind (which didn't like that busy, open-plan toilet block one bit)?

Of course, even the whole idea that body and mind are separate entities with a relationship with each other is just a concept, one that we are so used to hearing about that we have come to accept it as fact. It's a very Western idea, and we can trace it all the way back to – among others – the 17th-century French philosopher Descartes, who famously said, 'I think therefore I am', and after whom the 'Cartesian Split', a way of thinking of the clear division between mind and body, was named.

While it's true that this mind-body division is just one way of thinking about being human, it can actually be quite useful for birth – an event that can only be described as epic on both a physical and mental level. You can think about how much of an influential role your mind might play on your body during labour, and indeed, how the immense happenings in your body might also affect your mind.

Visualisations, affirmations, hippy vibrations?

As soon as you start talking about birth affirmations, or meditating your way through contractions, you're going to get a raised eyebrow. 'Oh yeah? Sounds like woo woo to me, take the epidural', some kind soul will say. So let's ditch the flowery birth talk for a while, and let's talk about what big tough athletes do when they're faced with an epic physical challenge. Oh, hang on a minute, guess what?! Yup, they use affirmations. Except they don't always call them that. Most often they call it, 'positive self-talk'. That sounds much more credible, right?

Yes, for years now, sports psychologists, Olympic medal-winners and top athletes from every area have been using the power of affirmations, mantras and visualisations – oh, sorry, 'positive self-talk' – knowing full well that where the mind goes, the body usually follows. Here are a few examples.

'I am the greatest!' Muhammad Ali was a pioneer when it came to knowing that expectations influenced reality. In fact, he even said, 'I am the greatest. I said that even before I knew I was.' He was even brave enough to use the word 'affirmation' – maybe they weren't so worried about woo woo in 1963, or were just too scared to correct him. 'It's the repetition of affirmations that leads to belief. And once that belief becomes a deep conviction, things begin to happen.' And my personal favourite quote from the greatest boxer that ever lived is this: 'If Ali says a mosquito can pull a plough, don't ask how. Hitch him up!'. In other words, if I say the impossible can be done, it will happen. Remember that one in transition.

'Why not me' At the 2012 Olympics, Canadian chef de mission Mark Tewkesbury had the whole team repeat this mantra to motivate and inspire them. 'Leave no stone unturned now because, I think when you get to the Games, the best place to be is, "I've done everything possible… why not me to win a medal, and when you get that kind of confidence and sureness, anything can happen', he said. So, make a plan. (See Being Birthzilla, pages 76 to 78.)

'You cannot be serious!' Tennis players – John McEnroe being a great example – will often repeat certain phrases on court, either under their breath or in a 'showy' way to the crowd, to motivate themselves and keep focused. Pete Sampras, who won 14 Grand Slam singles titles and is regarded as one of the greatest tennis players of all time, would say things like, 'Everything is OK', 'I need to let go of that last point and focus on the next point', and, 'I need to get aggressive with my feet'. Perfect for contractions, except maybe that last one about the feet.

'Hills are my friend' Marathon runners have a lot in common with labouring women: they have to keep focused on the finishing line even though it bloody well hurts for most of the race. If you google 'marathon mantras' you'll find hundreds, but here are a few from the top elite:

- 'This is what you came for' the mantra of Scott Jurek, an ultramarathon runner who used these words in 2010 when he set the US record for distance, running 165.7 miles in 24 hours.
- 'Think strong, be strong, finish strong.' Renée Metivier Baillie wrote this on her hand when she won the USATF 3,000 metres.
- 'Be water.' Olympic middle-distance runner Bolota Asmerom uses this Bruce Lee mantra to feel smooth but full of force.

Athletes don't just use positive self-talk, they also call on other psychological techniques, including:

Visualisation
Many athletes will spend time every day imagining various situations and positive outcomes in their head, to prepare their mind and think positive. Wayne Rooney finds out the colour of the opposing team's strip in advance so that he can picture himself scoring goals against them. Rugby champ Jonny Wilkinson uses visualisation on the pitch to help get the ball between the posts, 'I visualise the ball travelling

Ten Affirmations for Birth

Make these into posters for the wall of your birth room, or just repeat them in your mind or aloud during labour. Consider incorporating them into visualisations or meditations as you prepare for birth, and in doing so, create positive associations with the words in your mind and body.

It always seems impossible until it is done.

It's not pain, it's power.

Every surge brings me closer to my baby.

Soften. Open. Release.

I can and I will.

I am proud of my body and I trust it.

My body opens. My mind quiets. My baby descends.

I was born to do this.

Women all over the world are birthing with me.

My body knows how to give birth.

Not quite right? Make up your own! Or just nick one from an athlete. (I quite like 'Be water').

along that path and imagine the sensation of how the ball is going to feel when it hits my foot for the perfect strike', he says. And Andy Murray spends time sitting alone in a reserved Wimbledon centre court, focusing on past victories. All of them talk about the importance of making these visualisations really accurate, noticing every tiny detail – the smells, sounds and physical sensations of the experience they want to conquer.

> Spend just five minutes every day imagining your positive birth. Make it a part of your daily routine, perhaps each morning in the shower, or every night when you get into bed. Picture every small detail of the room you are in and the physical sensations you are having. Notice any smells and consider burning the same essential oil during your visualisations as you plan to use in your labour. Picture yourself coping brilliantly. Notice your breathing and try to take long slow breaths, in through the nose and out through the mouth, while you visualise. Consider adding a mantra and using the same one each day and in labour.

Meditation

It's all the rage in sports to borrow this technique from the world of yoga, and it's similar to visualisation, except it's about finding a state of inner calm and emptying your mind of… well, as much as you can, really! You don't need to be in a special place or physical position to meditate, although some pregnant women like to create a little 'birth altar' for themselves, with essential oils, positive affirmations, candles or flowers to help them focus. Then all you have to do is get comfortable, and either close your eyes or stare at a fixed object or point (like a candle flame). Focus on your breath without trying to change it, and accept your thoughts but at the same time allow them to float past rather than becoming fixed on them.

Psychologist Mihaly Csikszentmihalyi, author of *Finding Flow*, explains that many successful athletes will enter into a state that he calls 'flow' when they are performing well: a kind of meditative state where they are fully present in the moment and any sense of time is lost. This feeling, which athletes often call 'being in the zone', is experienced by all of us in moments that stand out; the 'flashes of intense living against the dull background of everyday living', as Csikszentmihalyi puts it.

Women in labour also talk about this state of 'flow', which some call 'Labour Land'. 'A labouring woman leaves her body and travels to the stars to collect the soul of her baby', a midwife once told me. The practice of meditation as you prepare for birth may well help you to prepare for what can feel like a very dream-like or spiritual journey to bring your baby into the world.

Reframing

This psychological technique involves looking at the same situation through a different 'frame', in order to transform the experience from negative to positive. It's not difficult to see why athletes, business people, actors and celebrities all use cognitive reframing to change and challenge the way they think. In some ways, you could argue that this whole book is an exercise in reframing, since it often asks you to look at something that you thought you 'had pegged' in a completely new way. You can use the technique of reframing in many ways as you prepare for birth, or in labour itself, for example:

Challenge your assumptions: take something you thought you knew about birth and ask, 'Why do I think this?' For example, if you have the thought that 'birth is the worst pain you can experience', ask yourself what evidence you have for this and how you know if it will be true for you. Then reframe it: 'birth will contain interesting and unexpected sensations and I have no idea what they will be like for me until I get there.'

Ask, 'What's good about this?': a contraction may feel tough, but what if you ask yourself, 'What's good about this?' Are there parts of it that feel interesting, fizzy, or sensual? Do you feel energised by it afterwards? Which parts of your body do not hurt at all, and what happens if you focus on them? What did you learn from the last contraction and how can it help you this time? What are you learning from this one?

Use different words: lots of the words around labour and birth are quite negative. By using more positive language, you might be able to change your expectations. Is it a contraction, a surge, an energy rush, a glow? Are you dilating, opening, unfolding, expanding? Find words that feel positive for you. (For more on this see page 86.)

'Choose the positive. You have choice, you are master of your attitude, choose the positive, the constructive. Optimism is a faith that leads to success.'   Bruce Lee

Fear and mental blocks

Many people, most notably Ina May Gaskin (see page 169), believe that fear in labour, or mental blocks, can actually physically prevent your labour from progressing. Gaskin tells stories of women she has attended in labour who have suddenly become fully dilated once they have spoken their fears aloud, or told their partner their truest and innermost thoughts. Given the power of the mind-body relationship, there's no reason why this shouldn't be true. I certainly feel that there was an element of 'holding on tight' involved when my body stubbornly refused to go into labour in my first pregnancy. In my next two pregnancies, I repeated the mantra, 'I am ready to let go,' once I had reached full term, visualising my cervix opening and bouncing on my birth ball as I did so. And I meant 'let go' in every sense; let go of my fears, let go of my everyday 'poise' and go to 'Labour Land', let go of my pregnancy, and let go of the baby held safe within me.

If you feel you have mental blocks, either as you prepare or while you are in labour, try different ways to release them, for example:

- Talk to someone, your partner or your friend, about how you really feel. Sit back-to-back or talk in the dark if this helps.
- Write a letter to your partner and tell them how you feel. Give it to them or just rip it up, the effect may be the same!
- Write a letter to your fears and tell them how you feel about them.
- Write a letter to your unborn baby and tell them any worries or feelings you have about the birth.
- Paint a picture, write a poem, or do something creative to express how you are feeling.
- Make a monument – go outside to a field, park or wood, and use 'found materials' like leaves, sticks, and stones to make something that represents your block. Spend time with it and either leave it or dismantle it as you see fit before you leave.
- Put on some favourite music and dance out your feelings. Let everything flow.

Your three brains

As well as considering the power of mind over matter, it's also interesting to learn a little bit about how the brain actually works, so that you can try to make this information work in your favour. I'm not going to start a lecture on neuroscience here, because how the brain works is actually pretty complicated. But, just as we've simplified things by imagining that humans are neatly split into a 'mind' and a 'body' that have a relationship with each other, we can also get some understanding about birth from thinking about the human brain in three simple sections.

The neocortex: This is the 'Boss brain', the 'thinking' part that remembers when you've run out of black olives. It's a new and modern bit of the brain, and it's what separates us out from animals in the sense that they don't normally vote on the *X Factor* or talk about Socrates.

The limbic brain: This is the 'mammalian' part of the brain, the 'feeling' brain. It's all about your emotions and largely operates at a subconscious level. It's very active when you're angry, scared, falling in love or yes, you guessed it, having a baby.

The cerebellum: This is the 'reptile' part of your brain, the 'doing' brain, and the very oldest bit. It just sits there and flicks its forked tongue in and out occasionally. It deals with basic questions like 'Will it eat me or can I eat it?', 'Shall I kill it or run?' and, 'If I kill it, can I eat it?'.

Life from the neck up

In these crazy modern times, we can become like little heads on sticks. We check our phones, we write our reports, we tap tap tap on our keyboards. We live a neocortical life, and can sometimes risk losing contact with our bodies below the neck. How do we feel? Many people are out of the habit of asking themselves this question, and feel cut off from their emotions, or too busy for them. What is going on in our bodies? We're not sure – is there an app for that?

So – giving birth. We make our plan. We read about how our foetus is developing week by week. We visit the MLU and talk about today's news stories or our partner and his new car with the friendly midwife. We purchase the right kind of car seat. The nursery is painted. And then… and then.

Labour time. It's like we've dived into the Cornish sea in a storm. There are huge waves, we are thrown onto all fours, the breath is knocked out of us, we gasp, we are making strange sounds, we are feeling extraordinary feelings. We are transported back through history and we are that earthy, hairy, unwashed, grunting cavewoman!

And then – oh my God! What does our partner think?! What does the midwife think?! We can't do this, it's just... embarrassing! Where the limbic, mammalian brain had begun to take hold, the neocortex steps in and says, 'No!' This is not how we do things round here! This gushing, guttural, groaning woman needs to be sanitised, normalised, and made to be quiet, please! And by the way, is there an app for that?!

Letting go

This is what Ina May Gaskin means when she says, 'let your monkey do it' (see page 171). We need to let go of inhibition, and of the thinking, planning, intellectualising part of our brain, when we give birth. For some this is harder than for others. If you think this will be a challenge for you, pregnancy is a great place to start. Any activity that gets you out of your head and into your body will help. Activities that get you to step out of your comfort zone are even better. Yoga, dance class, or just putting on music at home and really dancing, not how you

Sophie Fletcher, author of *Mindful Hypnobirthing*, tells us more...

Hypnobirthing uses all of the mind-body techniques you've read about in this chapter, designed and packaged up for pregnancy and birth. It's a crash course in birth psychology, teaching you how to reframe, visualise, and create a positive mindset around birth. All of the sports people mentioned in this section have actively used a mix of psychological techniques to improve performance, but what they really have in common is that they believe that they can do it and they actively learn how to. Many of them will have worked with their unconscious as well, taking steps to tackle that little voice we all have inside of us that that says 'Are you sure you can do it?' 'What if..?'. A hypnobirthing class helps guide you to a place where you know you can do it, deep down inside of you – and you have the tools to make it happen, both consciously and unconsciously.

What does it feel like? It feels lovely! A little bit like not being quite awake or asleep, and once you get used to it you may even think you are falling asleep. It's brilliant for women who struggle to sleep during pregnancy. Best of all – contrary to the myths – you are in control. You choose to do hypnosis, and how much you engage with it. I can never make someone do something they don't want to do.

Hypnobirthing is not just about relaxed, calm, pain-free birth – it's about creating strength, belief and resilience so that whatever journey your birth takes, you have the techniques to help you get into the headspace to make the right choices and decisions for you and your baby. I even work with preparing women for positive caesarean births. In my experience a hypnobirth can be a home water birth, an induction or a caesarean – but it's always a positive experience.

Try this easy hypnobirthing technique (also used by Andy Murray!). It's called 'Creating an Anchor': Think of a moment in time where you have felt really good about yourself, strong, focused, happy – you choose. Importantly it has to be the actual moment you felt great, not just before or just after, the actual moment! Close your eyes, take some deep breaths to relax yourself and imagine it, as if it were happening again. When you get that rush of good feelings just squeeze your thumb and forefinger together. Imagine all those positive feelings collecting there. Repeat this action about five times, letting that feeling get stronger and stronger. Whenever you are in a situation where you want to bring back that feeling, all you have to do is squeeze your thumb and forefinger together. You have made a link between mind and body! Easy, isn't it?!

You can download an MP3 for free at **mindful-hypnobirthing.co.uk** and have a go at a typical hypnosis preparation track.

think you should be dancing (shut up neocortex!), but how you would dance if you were a monkey or a three-year-old and really didn't give a shit. Get down and get dirty, and get ready to let go.

Hypnobirthing

Hypnobirthing, or birth hypnosis, is a great way of getting some structured input into your personal mind-body relationship. A hypnobirthing teacher will work with you, often one-to-one, to give you techniques to overcome fear and stay calm and focused in your labour. You can also get hypnobirthing downloads, CDs or books. There are several different birth hypnosis providers listed in the Resources.

Exercise in pregnancy

Pregnant women have for a long time been considered delicate flowers, ineligible for even mildly strenuous effort and excluded, not only from contact sports, but even from many party activities including blowing up balloons and dancing the *Hokey Cokey*. But this perception of 'pregnancy as weakness' is finally being challenged, and I think it's actually really psychologically important that women realise what a time of great strength and vitality pregnancy can be.

Of course, if exercise to you means prising the lid off the biscuit tin, then that's your choice, but it's worth remembering that eating a healthy balanced diet in pregnancy (which can of course include

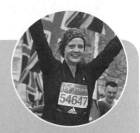

Emma Bateman ran several miles, four times a week until she was eight months pregnant. After that, she slowed to a walk.

I started running two years after the birth of my first child, when a friend and then my GP finally helped me confront the fact that I'd had serious PND and depression more generally. Running became a critical part of my physical and mental health self-care plan. I was running four times a week, every week, and had completed a couple of half marathons.

So when I got pregnant the second time, it was critically important to me to keep running. I genuinely think I would have lost the plot without it. I don't like swimming, yoga etc, and can't bear the thought of exercising with other people in a class. I love the solitude of running.

Throughout my pregnancy I ran four times a week every week (three short runs of 3–4 miles and one longer one up to about 7–8 miles at the weekends) until I was about eight months, at which point it felt uncomfortable so I walked the same distances each day instead.

I worked full-time until I went into labour, so running/ walking was a huge part of my personal, emotional and physical resilience – keeping me fit, but also getting me out into the fresh air every day and giving me space and time to escape. Running also kept my weight sensible and helped me sleep better at night.

I checked with my midwife and doula, who both agreed that I should run for as long as I wanted to and felt comfortable to. I wore decent trainers to protect my posture, but other than that made no adjustments at all. I also got lots of brilliant strong support from the Run Mummy Run community online, where I found loads of pregnant women who run. Some people told me not to run, or shouted lovely offensive things at me in the street, but actually when I saw my reflection running with my bump, I felt strong and proud – just like when I gave birth.

I went for a natural labour and definitely felt that my physical and emotional strength from running were incredibly useful (in fact, many of my birthing and running visualisations and affirmations are the same!)

After the birth, I didn't do any exercise for six weeks, but then gradually built up again through walking and then running, and started training properly again. I ran the Birmingham half marathon six months after my daughter was born and my first-ever marathon (London) just before her first birthday, which I had always had in mind as a personal goal, to prove to myself that I could do it.

moments of indulgence!) is better for both you and your baby, and that health complications such as gestational diabetes are more common if you are overweight or obese.

All of the current advice on exercise in pregnancy offers a similar message: listen to your body. If you have never exercised before or are very unfit, don't launch into a hardcore fitness programme in the first trimester. As you would normally, build up slowly, and if you find yourself breathless or experiencing any kind of pain or discomfort, stop.

If you were already exercising regularly before you got pregnant, you can carry on with the same routine, but again, listen to your body, and speak to your fitness instructor or midwife if you have any concerns.

Evidence-based birth choices

You might be familiar with the idea of making decisions in pregnancy or labour that are 'evidence-based'. This generally means that the decision is founded on the best research that has been done on the topic. For example, if you are going to be induced because you are 42 years old and have been told that it's not recommended that you go past 40 weeks pregnant, you want to know how your doctor or midwife knows this to be true.

You want to know that somebody, somewhere has looked into this and studied loads of knackered old pregnant women like you and worked out that induction definitely is the safest and best decision you can make.

You want to know that their recommendation has an 'evidence base'. In other words, that their house of advice is build on sturdy and robust foundations. It's not just a random opinion. Make sense?

Of course, if there really was just a nice kindly boffin somewhere, studying a group of 40-something preggos and noting on his clipboard why the 50 per cent who got induced had a fabbydabby birth and the other half all died an unspeakable death, then this whole evidence-based birth thing would be super simple. Clear cut, black and white, and really, really helpful.

Unfortunately, it's a bit more complicated than that. The fact is, there are kindly boffins all over the world researching every angle of pregnancy and birth on a regular basis. This research is conducted in different ways, with different sized groups of people, in different parts of the world, in different decades of history. Some of this research may ask one question – for example, do we get a better outcome for the baby when we induce women over 40? – but not ask another question – for example, did the women in the study know their midwife or not? So we won't ever know if those women who had poor outcomes in that particular study might have had better outcomes if they had been looked after by someone they had met before, and whom they really trusted.

In other words, all evidence is created equal, but some is more equal than others. The Royal College of Obstetricians and Gynaecologists (RCOG) deals with this by grading their guidelines according to how strong the evidence they are based on actually is. Grade A, for example, is what they consider to be top-quality evidence, usually based on something called a Randomised Controlled Trial (RCT) – that's where similar people get different interventions (or none) and the results are compared. Grades B and C are based on less strong evidence, like reviews of the existing literature on a topic, and Grade D is given to guidelines based on case reports and expert opinion.

Shockingly, only about 9 per cent of the RCOG guidelines are based on Grade A evidence! And even more shockingly, only about 50 per cent of their guidelines are based on Grade B, C and D evidence! Hang on a mo, I hear you say, that leaves about 40 per cent of their guidelines unaccounted for. What evidence are they based on?! Here's a revelation for you. They're not based on any evidence. Forty per cent of the guidelines are based on the recommendations of the people who develop the guidelines, according to their clinical experience. In other words, they are based on opinion, not evidence.

The reason I'm taking you on this slightly complex tour through the workings of the RCOG is to get across a wider point: even the top experts in birth and evidence don't have all the answers. If you're pregnant, it's important to keep asking questions of your care providers, to try to find out on what evidence they are basing the advice they are giving you. It's also important to know that even if the advice is based on a particular piece of evidence, it doesn't automatically mean that that evidence is top quality. And it's also possible that the advice you are being given is based on no evidence at all, just personal opinion.

Of course, just because we don't have the research to back up our opinion, doesn't make it automatically wrong either. Midwives and obstetricians who spend their working lives dealing with labouring women will have a huge amount of knowledge and lived experience that we need to respect and trust. In emergency situations in particular, we will always be glad to be in their capable hands. But if there is not an emergency, it's really OK to ask questions and do your own research on your options.

When making pregnancy choices, it can be really hard to get a clear picture or decide on the 'right' course of action. There is rarely a situation that is black and white. Even if there is a really robust study about your particular dilemma, that study didn't include a very important person – you! Every woman is different. You might be over 40 and in the pink of health, really physically fit, totally confident in your body and in a geographical area that offers one-to-one midwifery care. Or you might be over 40, obese, diabetic and really worried about giving birth in your local overstretched obstetric unit. You need to think about your own personal circumstances, and also factor in how you intuitively feel about this birth in your heart of hearts. That's not very evidence based, you might say; but then again, neither are some of the RCOG guidelines.

If you want to take a look at some of the evidence for yourself, here are some suggestions for good resources.

Your healthcare provider. The person recommending a certain course of action should be able to point you to the evidence upon which this suggestion is based.

> **'Giving birth is a life-changing event. The care that a woman receives during labour has the potential to affect her – both physically and emotionally, in the short and longer term – and the health of her baby. Good communication, support and compassion from staff, and having her wishes respected, can help her feel in control of what is happening and contribute to making birth a positive experience for the woman and her birth companion(s).'**
>
> **Extract from the Introduction to NICE Clinical Guideline 190**

NICE guidelines. These guidelines are put together by teams of academics, professionals and service users, are based on the best available evidence, and are regularly reviewed and revised. NICE is a UK public body and part of the Department of Health; however, practitioners in many other parts of the world look to NICE to find the best standards of practice, so, if you are reading this book and are beyond the UK, you may still find NICE guidelines useful and highly applicable to your situation. Particularly useful is CG190. Search for 'NICE CG190' or search for 'NICE guideline _____' and fill in the blank with the issue you need more information about. Alternatively visit **rcog.org.uk/guidelines** and use their search box – select NICE guidelines in the dropdown menu.

Cochrane reviews. Cochrane reviews are internationally recognised as the highest standard in evidence-based healthcare resources. Search for 'Cochrane review _____' and fill in the blank with the issue you want to know more about, for example 'Cochrane review induction of labour'. Alternatively visit **cochranelibrary.com** and use the search box.

RCOG Green-top Guidelines. Guidelines for UK obstetricians on pretty much every pregnancy and birth scenario. Visit www.rcog.org. uk/guidelines and use their brilliant search facility, either to search the Green-top Guidelines, or to explore the dropdown menu to find other guidelines and reports, including the NICE guidelines.

ACOG and SOGC. The American College of Obstetricians and Gynaecologists (ACOG) and the Society of Obstetricians and Gynaecologists of Canada (SOGC) have practice bulletins and guidelines that can be found at **acog.org/Resources-And-Publications/Practice-Bulletins-List** and **jogc.com/clinical-practice-guidelines** respectively.

Which? Birth Choice. Want to know how your local hospital compares to the national average when it comes to everything from numbers of caesareans to your chances of having stitches? Find information about where to give birth and a wide range of stats on all of your nearest units, searchable by postcode, at **which.co.uk/birth-choice**.

Evidence Based Birth. This American website, written by researcher Rebecca Dekker, gives a really accessible overview of the evidence relating to many of the major birth choices and dilemmas. **evidencebasedbirth.com**

You can find more sources of information in the Resources at the back of this book.

Continuity of care

This has to be the most boring and unsexy title for something that can actually have a massive impact on the kind of birth experience you end up having. 'Continuity of care' simply means, 'knowing your midwife'. The researchers discuss endlessly what they think continuity of care means, or ought to mean – but I think I already know – don't you? When I'm all naked and grunty and leaky and maybe a little bit scared, I kind of want to be in a room with people I feel utterly safe with. And that means – for me anyway – my partner, and just one, or maybe two, midwives, who I've met before several times and who I really like, and trust. Simples.

The evidence on continuity of care is clear. Women have better births, with higher levels of satisfaction, and better outcomes, when they know their midwife. Birth is safer this way. And midwives often prefer it too, because they get to really connect with the women they care for and not feel like they are just a tiny cog in a big meaningless machine.

Some of the research stats on continuity are amazing. Women who are cared for by a midwife they know have fewer caesareans and are more likely to give birth vaginally without intervention. They have higher levels of satisfaction, are more positive about their overall birth experience, and feel less anxious and more in control. They are also:

- 24% less likely to experience pre-term birth
- 16% less likely to lose their baby
- 15% less likely to have an epidural
- 16% less likely to have an episiotomy

This information is great – but what can you do with it?
Unfortunately, although we have a lot of evidence that continuity of care has a really positive impact, for many women it is a long way

from their birth experience. In reality, many women have never met the midwife who attends them in birth, and often, due to shift changes, will meet two or more new faces during their labour and birth experience. Armed with the knowledge that this might not be the optimal care for women in labour, you could:

Get a doula. A doula can provide you with continuous support through pregnancy and birth. (More info on page 153.)

Hire an independent midwife (IM). A fully qualified IM will bring the relationship-based care you are probably craving. (See page 154.)

Ask for continuity. Tell your local midwifery team that having a relationship with your midwife before the day you give birth is very important to you. It's possible they might find a way to make it happen, and if not, your feedback may encourage them to improve the system for future women.

Write to or tweet your MP. Let your MP know that you would like to know your midwife! Again, being vocal about what matters to you in childbirth may help women in the future, even if it doesn't directly help you.

Watch out for NHS changes. Recently a big review of UK maternity care took place, known as Better Births. The reviewers were well aware of the positive impact of a known midwife, and, as a result, initiatives like a personal 'maternity budget' may be rolled out nationally, meaning you can vote for continuity of care with your wallet.

More about... doulas

Doulas are a new-fangled trend, but a very, very old idea. They are simply women who 'mother the mother', who nurture women in pregnancy, comfort them in birth, and care for them in the days and weeks that follow.

In our current over-stretched maternity system, many women are not getting the continuity of care that has been proven by swathes of research to have such a beneficial impact on both the safety and the experience of giving birth. If you want to be sure you obtain this, you may wish to hire an independent midwife (see next section), but an alternative (and cheaper option) is to find a doula.

You will usually hire your doula during pregnancy and she will spend time with you talking about your plans and hopes for birth. It's really important that you 'click' with your doula, since the human element of connection is the vital ingredient here. As you prepare for birth, your doula should listen to you and respect your choices. She's not a medical professional; she can't deliver babies or administer medical procedures. Her role is to simply make you feel like a goddess, no matter where or how you want to or have to give birth.

Doulas can also 'advocate' for you, making sure that your birth plan or wishes are listened to and kept in mind, and that you are treated at all times with respect and dignity. Letting a doula take this role can be a real relief for dads, freeing them up to enjoy the birth of their child without having to worry about liaising with professionals or understanding the ins and outs of hospital protocol.

Doulas are a 'paid extra' of course, costing from £200 for a less experienced doula up to £600+ for a doula who has attended many births, although it may cost more in cities. This includes working with you before the birth, being on call for your labour and staying with you throughout – no matter how long this might be – and supporting you afterwards with follow-up visits. A 'postnatal doula' will come and look after you in the first few weeks of your baby's life and help with everything from sleep and feeding issues to the washing up.

What is an Independent Midwife?

If I told you that for between £2,000 and £5,000, you could have your own personal midwife, caring for you and championing your choices, wherever or however you decide to have your baby, your immediate response might be that it's simply too expensive. But hold on – don't some people spend similar amounts on cars, wedding dresses, or the annual holiday?

Some would argue that getting an IM is a financial priority worth making. On the other hand, money is tight. Some of us can't afford a nice car, or a wedding, or a hotel with a poolside bar, so paying out for something we can all get for free in the UK – midwifery care – might seem ridiculous. But this book is all about informing you of your choices, so before you skip to the next section, bear with me while I tell you a little bit about why those women who do fork out for an independent midwife usually describe it as the best money they've ever spent.

An independent midwife is a fully trained and qualified midwife who works outside the NHS in a self-employed capacity. It's this 'self-employed' nature that makes IMs truly autonomous and unique – and it's important to stress that when I talk about IMs in this book I'm referring to these self-employed midwives, who belong to the organisation IMUK, and not any other private midwifery companies or provisions.

An IM will offer you exactly the same antenatal and postnatal clinical care as you would receive under the NHS; for example, she will monitor blood pressure, urine and foetal well-being at every antenatal appointment.

All of these appointments will take place in your home and your midwife will come, often with books, gifts and plenty of cake. Other days you will provide the gifts and cake and you will sit and talk at length over tea and do what women do best: empathise, giggle, chatter, connect.

This awesome woman will become your rock. She will listen to you and talk you through your fears. She will be there for you whenever you need her, and as the birth approaches, she will visit more and more frequently and fill you with confidence and excitement about what is to come. You will eat more cake. You will laugh more. And then, one night, you will get a little niggle at 3am, and you will text her, and if you want her to come, she will come. Once you are in labour, she will be there for you whether it last three hours or three days, and no matter how it unfolds.

IMs provide the kind of 'continuity of care' that has been shown in many studies to make birth both a more enjoyable experience and a safer one. Most IMs work outside the NHS because they have a strong belief in women's innate ability to birth beautifully that they do not feel is always supported in the current system. They often attend home births and they can be a godsend if you fall into a 'higher risk' category such as breech, twins or VBAC, as they are able to take time to assess the whole picture and give you personalised care. But IMs are not 'mavericks' – like all UK midwives they are registered with and regulated by the Nursing and Midwifery Council (NMC) and, should you genuinely need obstetric care, they will refer you for it and support you throughout.

Postnatally, IMs will give you a gold standard experience that most NHS midwives simply will not have time for. They will be there, in

'Because I know you': the power of continuity of care

During my third birth I had a lot of doubt. (I am a born worrier.) My second baby had been big at 10lb 4oz and I couldn't shake the idea that I had grown a monster for this third birth. Towards the end of labour (probably during transition), I really felt panicked and like something might be wrong. A few minutes later, my baby boy (slightly smaller at 9lb 11oz) was safely in my arms.

At one of my many postnatal visits with my IM, I asked her, 'Tara, how did you know it was going to be alright? I mean, how did you really... know?'

'Because I know you', she replied. 'All those antenatal visits, you build up a picture, a picture of what is "normal", not normal for any old woman, but normal for Milli. You learn what Milli's skin tone looks like when she is vital and happy. You record her blood pressure and get an insight into what the parameters of normal are there. You learn about Milli's voice, her physicality, her breathing – what she's like in every way when all is well. And if anything deviates even slightly from that, you can see it, right away, quite clearly.'

We sat in contented silence and I felt the deep sense of reassurance that comes from knowing somebody really genuinely gives a shit about you and has your back. This is the confidence and mutual trust that comes from the kind of human, relationship-based care that IMs offer. For me, worth every penny.

Every woman deserves this kind of midwifery care.

person and usually any time you need to text or phone them, through the first days and weeks, helping you with feeding, taking time to debrief your birth experience and making sure you recover and start motherhood feeling great. There will be plenty more cake at this stage, too.

If you think you'd like an IM, you'll need to find your nearest and meet with them – it's extremely important that you 'click' because in this situation, the relationship is the vital ingredient. If you are not sure you can afford an IM, you may be able to spread your payments, or, in cases of hardship, their fee may be reduced. Some have even been known to barter: one IM exchanged her services for a fairly substantial amount of hairdressing, I'm told.

 At the time of writing, independent midwives are challenging a ruling from the NMC that their insurance provision for attending births is inadequate. This situation is evolving rapidly and different IMs in different geographical areas are finding different solutions until a resolution is found at a national level. If you want to consider booking an IM for your intrapartum care, find your nearest on the IMUK website (see Resources) and ask them to update you on the current situation.

What about water birth?

When they step over the edge of the birth pool and lower their mahoosively pregnant body down into the deep warm water, most women say one thing, and one thing only: 'Ahhhhhhh'. This deep sigh has a double meaning: 'Ahhh, this feels so blimmin' good I could cry with happiness', and 'Ahhh, I get it now'.

It's impossible to describe just how brilliant water birth is and how great it feels: you'll just have to trust me. I've done it twice. It's often described as 'a form of pain relief', but there is much, much more to it than this.

Yes, it's true that something – maybe the warmth of the water (much deeper and wider than a conventional bath) – takes the edge off birth contractions. Several different studies have shown that women who have water births report lower levels of pain and use less pain medication than their counterparts on land. Other studies show that you are less likely to tear in water, perhaps due to the counter-pressure of the water on your perineum.

Of course, water is supportive to your whole body, which can be a huge relief in the final stages of pregnancy, a time when most women feel heavy and cumbersome. In the water, suddenly you have a freedom of movement and this can also help with comfort levels: if you want to quickly shift positions, you can.

Perhaps water birth is also less painful because you feel more protected by the 'big dark skirts' of the birth pool. You have more privacy, and you are harder to reach – if anyone wants to touch you or examine you, they have to ask nicely, or get wet, or possibly both. This feeling of protection and privacy surely helps oxytocin levels, which in turn keep labour progressing and make us feel happy and loved.

Perhaps women who choose water birth are also more likely to enjoy labour because of their mindset. Water birth is a conscious positive choice. Anyone who gets in a birth pool is making a statement: 'I want my birth to be a certain kind of birth, and I'm prepared to go to certain lengths to make it that way'. They are saying, 'Hold the epidural, I want to be mobile, conscious, and active'.

Whether it's positive mental attitude, feelings of privacy and protection offered by the water, easier mobility or just a nice big hot bath, water birth works. Here's what a few women had to say about its magical effect:

'It helped me stay private and protected from the anxiety of being poked or prodded. I felt hidden and sheltered and able to get on with the job at hand instead of worrying about anyone touching me/looking at my bottom half!!!! Oh and the pain relief compared with my two on land births was fantastic, I didn't need any gas and air or anything. Best thing to do in labour is to get in water!!' Rachel Nolan

'The best experience I could've hoped for. Took the weight of my belly away and I was able to move around as I wanted. The water felt so soothing and relaxing. I would do it again in a heartbeat.' Nikki Jones

'It was comforting, warming and relaxing. My partner was feeding me strawberries between contractions. A great experience.' Susie Heywood

'It was just wonderful – I felt weightless and the warmth of the water felt so soothing. There was no way that I was getting out of there! I had no tears or grazes, which perhaps was a combo of the gentle pushing and the water.' Marika Hart

'As the water took my weight it gave me the freedom to move and it really took the edge off the pain, it was so soothing. I believe it allowed me to experience 'foetal ejection' so I didn't even consciously push – my body took over and in three intense contractions my little one made her way into the world. I didn't even try, it was amazing!' Kelly Delaney

Water Birth FAQs

Can I have a water birth in hospital?

If you really, really want a water birth, home is the place you are most likely to get one. Not all units have pools and sometimes the ones that do have practical issues that mean the pool is not available. In some cases, women have been known to take their own pool, but this is rare and must be negotiated with your unit. Talk to your care providers and find out what your water birth chances and options are in your local area.

Where do I get a pool for a home birth?

You can buy a pool online or hire one. Second-hand or borrowed pools are fine but you will need to buy a new liner. Some home birth support groups, PBM groups or local doulas and midwives will lend or hire birth pools too.

How long does it take to fill the pool?

This depends on your water system. If you have constant hot water, it will be considerably quicker than if you have to heat a tank, add this to the pool, cover, and wait for the next tank to heat. In all cases it's best to start filling the pool at the tiniest twinge of labour – the worst case scenario is that it's a false alarm and you will just get to have a big bath, rather than a big birth, that day!

Why doesn't the baby breathe underwater?

A baby does not take their first breath until they are born and in some ways, the water of the pool 'tricks' baby into waiting a little longer before they take this breath. Something called the 'dive reflex' means that the 'glottis' at the back of the throat will stay closed while the baby is underwater. Newborn lungs are also already filled with fluid, making it almost impossible for the water from the pool to enter their lungs. Finally, prostaglandin levels in the baby take a few moments to drop at birth, making the first breath possible. Until you bring your baby to the surface, they will be getting their oxygen supply from the placenta, just as they have while 'underwater' in the amniotic fluid of your womb.

How deep should the water be?

It's really important that the water is deep enough for your bottom to remain fully submersed during the birth. This is because, if the baby is partly born and they come up from under the water, they could be triggered into taking their first breath. You also need at least 18 inches of water to get the full benefits of buoyancy – that lovely feeling of weightlessness that feels so good.

When can I get in the pool?

This is a matter for some debate. Some women are told not to get into the pool in early labour, in case the warm relaxation of the water slows their labour. However, women who call the hospital in early labour are often also advised to have a bath – confusing, huh?! My advice? If you you want to get in, get in. If it slows your labour or stalls it completely, maybe this is what you need. Have a rest, and fear not; your labour will get going again at some point, and you will meet your baby soon and when you are both ready.

What temperature should the water be?

Make sure you monitor the water temperature and keep it around 32 to 38 Celsius. Use your own judgement too: if it feels too hot or too cold, it probably is.

What should I wear for a water birth?

Wear what you feel comfortable in. For some, that's simply your Birthday Suit. Midwives have seen it all before and won't bat an eyelid at your naked body. Others prefer to wear a bra or even a bikini, although you're going to have to take the bottom half off at some point, obviously.

Can my partner get in with me?

Yes, but only if you want them to. It's your party.

Do I have to get out to be monitored or examined?

You shouldn't 'have to' do anything in labour that you don't want to do. Vaginal exams to check dilation are optional for all women, regardless of whether they are having a water birth, and if your labour is cracking on (and trust me, you'll know when it is), there isn't really a desperate need to know your dilation. Midwives can also check dilation using the 'purple line' method – as you become more dilated a purple line will appear in your coccyx area – ask your midwife if they know how to do this (see page 94). Midwives should also be able to monitor your baby's heartbeat using an underwater Doppler, and they should do this between contractions and with minimum disturbance to you as you labour. If your labour seems to be stalling or something doesn't feel right, you might like to get out of the pool to be checked, and also to see if moving on dry land changes the dynamics for the better.

If my baby is born in water, when should I get out?
As long as everyone is happy and healthy, there's no rush. Some like to stay in the pool, cord attached, while they say hello to their baby. Often this is the moment when partners or even young siblings like to get in and meet the new family member! It's a lovely way to make a gentle transition from womb to world and begin enjoying skin-to-skin. Some women also deliver the placenta in the pool, although not all midwives will be up for this, and it's worth talking to them in advance if you think you might like to do so.

What about the microbiome, how does water birth affect this?
The short answer is, we just don't know. Some wonder if being 'washed' at birth could have a detrimental effect on the development of the baby's microbiome, but as you will see in the full section on the microbiome on page 165, there is a great deal that we don't understand about this developing field of science. If you are worried about this, remember that there are other ways to boost the seeding of the microbiome, like skin-to-skin contact and breastfeeding. You could also choose to get out just before you deliver, although be warned, when this is actually suggested, you may be heard to say, 'I don't give a s**t about the micro-f***ing-biome, I'm not getting out of this pool!'

Are there any reasons why I can't have a water birth?
Women are discouraged from water birth if they have risk factors, such as twins, high BMI, previous caesarean, or other complications. However, women with twins, high BMI, previous caesareans and more have all given birth in water! If you want a water birth, but find barriers are being put up, talk to your healthcare providers and ask for support from your supervisor of midwives. You can also benefit from talking to other women who have been in similar positions, and social media support groups can be an excellent place to find them. You may also find that an independent midwife will support your water birth choice if NHS midwives are unable to do so.

The 'quickening': feeling your baby move

You know that moment when you first feel a little tickle inside, a little flutter of butterfly wings, and you wonder, was it something I ate? Is there a bee up my shirt? Or was that... could it have been... no way! That was my baby moving!!!

Turns out this super-exciting moment in every pregnancy has a name from days of yore: it's called the 'quickening'. Taking its origin from the word 'quick' meaning 'alive', this would have been the time from which an unborn child was considered to be living, long before we peed on sticks and waited for blue lines, or saw our in utero offspring frolic on hospital scanners.

If this is your first baby, you'll probably feel the first movements sometime around 18 to 20 weeks, and in subsequent pregnancies it'll be a bit earlier, due to the slightly softer and saggier nature of your uterus (yes, even that part of you is softer and saggier these days).

So the first movements are called the quickening, and it's perhaps no coincidence that this word looks like the perfect title for a horror movie, because things can get pretty weird after this. The days of sighing and placing a loving hand on your belly as your baby flutters secretively inside you don't last long – before you know it your inner butterfly will metamorphose into what can feel like a giant caterpillar wearing hobnail boots. By the later weeks of pregnancy, you'll be able to lie back on the sofa and watch your bump ripple and leap as if you'd swallowed a litter of Great Danes.

Aside from the comedy mileage in scaring childless friends in the pub with a quick game of 'Kick off the Beer Mat', there's a serious side to foetal movements. Being in tune with your baby's activity is a vital way of monitoring their wellbeing. The charity Mama Academy recommends the following:

- Your baby should have a regular pattern of movements from around 24 weeks. Keep track of your baby's daily activity, and if you think that anything has changed, don't wait to report it – phone your maternity unit and get checked without delay.
- If you are unsure whether your baby has moved because you are having a busy day, lie on your left side and concentrate on their movements for up to an hour. Don't wait any longer than this, even if you are still not sure.
- Don't rely on hand-held monitors, phone apps or Dopplers at home to check your baby's heartbeat. Even if they detect a heartbeat, this

doesn't mean your baby is well and you may be falsely reassured.

* Remember, it is not true that babies' movements slow down or stop towards the end of pregnancy. If you think your baby's movements have changed in any way, call your maternity unit immediately.

Above all, be insistent if you feel something is not right. You are the mother and you know best, so if you are at all concerned, make sure you get checked and if necessary ask for a second or even third opinion.

Finding out the sex... or not

It's a dilemma most modern couples face that would have been unthinkable just a few decades ago: is it better to find out the sex so you can plan ahead, or is there something to be said for the air of mystery that waiting until the 'birth-day' affords? And then there's the argument that gender has become just another way of 'pigeon-holing' people anyway, and that the less focus we give it, the better.

Regardless of this, you might feel you simply cannot stand the suspense, and want to find out at the 20-week scan, giving you a practical head-start if you want to purchase gender-specific baby items, and, according to some, making you feel more connected to your unborn child once you can imagine their sex or even name them.

If you find out in advance, you might like to take this exciting moment to a whole new level with a 'gender reveal party'. Parents-to-be ask the sonographer to write the baby's sex secretly on a piece of paper. Then a cake is baked that is 'colour coded' (usually pink or blue)

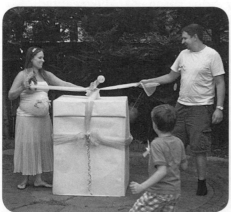
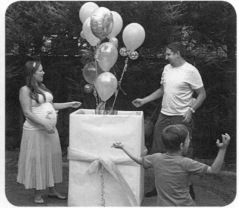

on the inside, and this is cut by mum and dad surrounded by friends and family.

As well as the cake, there are other creative ideas for the moment of discovery. Gemma Cash, from Essex, paid a balloon company to fill an enormous box with pink or blue balloons for her gender reveal party. 'We bought special party wear, and decorated everywhere appropriately, we made pink or blue ribbon badges so that all our guests could choose which sex they thought the baby would be. Then we called all our guests out to the garden for the big reveal.

'My husband and I opened the box together and discovered the sex of our baby surrounded by our children, friends and family. Looking back I think it was a really special way to find out, and best of all is having ours and our children's reactions captured on camera, to show to our little boy when he is older.'

Feeling disappointed about gender

It's really hard to talk about any feelings of negativity or disappointment around pregnancy, birth or motherhood; it's all supposed to be wall-to-wall joy. But while some love finding out the gender at the scan, other women secretly admit that they felt upset or even devastated when they found out they weren't going to be having the little girl or little boy they were hoping for. This could be an argument in favour of waiting till the birth to find out, when you're likely to be overwhelmed with emotion and therefore less likely to care about such minor details.

'I know parents who have had a really strong desire one way or another, and have been crying at their scan because they didn't get what they wanted!' says midwife Hannah Roe. 'But I've never had a parent cry at the birth because they didn't get the sex they wanted!'

Because of these experiences, Hannah decided not to find out the gender at her 20-week scan in either of her own pregnancies.

'Not knowing what I was having really helped me through both my labours, it was that thing that I focused on and it helped me to concentrate. In my recent, second birth, my husband was really hoping for a son, and for me to be able to lift him out of the water and say "It's a boy!" was just the best feeling ever – I felt elated and so proud.'

If you want to discover the sex of your baby yourself, make sure you put this in your birth plan (see page 104).

Can scans be wrong about gender?

It's highly unlikely and unusual, but it does very, very occasionally happen. Here's a cautionary tale:

'One family I knew got a big surprise. The sonographer was absolutely certain the baby was a girl, and they spent the rest of the pregnancy bonding with the bump called Rose. The dresses were bought. The room painted pink. So when the baby was born, no one checked the gender. Much later the midwife asked if the baby had a name yet and they said with pride "Yes, Rose". To which the midwife asked awkwardly how that should be spelt. That's when she broke it to them that they needed to take a look. The baby is now called Rob.' Sabrina Gant, hypnobirthing teacher

All about... the microbiome

Breaking news: vaginas may play a key role in childbirth. Yes folks, you heard it here first. As shocking as it may sound, researchers are discovering that, rather than just being an optional and at times rather problematic exit route, the humble birth canal might actually be fundamentally important to the future health and wellbeing of our babies, and our species.

Researchers on the Human Microbiome Program at New York University (NYU) School of Medicine have actually been swabbing newborn caesarean babies with gauze that's been incubated in the mother's vagina, and inspired by this, some caesarean mums have followed suit, rubbing their baby with vaginal juices immediately after they are born.

Did some of you say 'yuck'? Yes, I thought you would – because we've all been taught that bottoms are dirty, germs are bad, and vaginas – well, let's not even go there with the things we've been taught about them. But stay with me – because what I'm about to explain will challenge the way you think, and not just about bottoms.

Scientists are only just beginning to understand the microbiome – the unique colony of bacteria that populates every human – and they're looking into the role it plays, not just in birth, but in every aspect of our mental and physical health. So cutting edge is this field that some refer to the microbiome as a 'newly discovered organ', and believe that further understanding of it may throw light on some facets of humanity: disease, personality, life expectancy, and more.

As a baby is born vaginally, the colonisation of the baby's microbiome begins. In fact, studies of the birth canal have shown that in the time before labour starts, the make-up of vaginal bacteria changes, for example to include extra Lactobacillus, a bacteria that aids in the digestion of milk. Studies comparing the microbiomes of vaginally-born babies with those born via caesarean have shown differences in their gut bacteria as long as seven years after delivery.

There is much we don't yet understand about why, or how much these differences may matter. But scientists are beginning to explore connections between the microbiome of caesarean-born babies and the rising incidence of health problems such as obesity, asthma, eczema, and type 1 diabetes.

Dr Maria Gloria Dominguez-Bello, an associate professor in the Human Microbiome Program at the NYU School of Medicine, is investigating whether we can help replace the colonisation of the microbiome 'manually', allowing caesarean-born babies to have the same beneficial start in life. This is done quite simply: a gauze is placed in the vagina, left for one hour, and removed just before the birth by caesarean, then rubbed on the mouth, face and body of the newborn baby.

What Dominguez-Bello has found so far – and her research is still in the early stages – is that this process does make a difference to the microbiome of the newborn, but that it is not as effective in the process of colonisation as simply being born vaginally.

'When we analyzed the sharing, we doubled the number of bacteria that the C-section babies were exposed to. But the vaginal process was six times as much. So the vaginal delivery still exposes the baby to a lot more. That's logical because during labour, the baby is rubbing against the mucosa of the birth canal for a long time and bacteria start growing even before the baby is out — growing and colonizing the baby during birth. Also, C-sections involve antibiotics, and we don't know what the effect is of that gram of penicillin.'

Research like this can be problematic to discuss because it raises the 'vaginal birth is better' issue, but, argues Dominguez-Bello, whose findings form a key part of the film *Microbirth*, while we need to accept that medical interventions can save lives, we also need to make sure they are completely necessary.

'The problem is thinking that there's no cost. And so far, the point is, both moms and most doctors think there is absolutely no cost of C-sections, C-sections are okay. And we still don't understand what the risk is. We haven't quantified it in proper studies, it's all

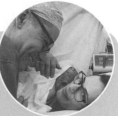

Our Seeding Story: Frederique Rattue was one of the first-ever UK mums to seed her baby's microbiome in February 2015.

When I learned that I would have to have my fourth baby by caesarean, I was initially sorry that I would not be able to give him the same start in life as my other three children who were born vaginally. I had seen the film *Microbirth*, and read about the research at NYU and how they were swabbing babies with vaginal bacteria after caesarean and finding they have more similar microbiomes to babies born vaginally.

I asked my team at St Helier Hospital in Carshalton – supervisor of midwives, Maria Mills Shaw, and obstetrician Mr Adetunji Matiluko – if they would support me in the seeding process. Together with them I planned a 'woman-centred caesarean', with the seeding of my baby's microbiome incorporated. I feel glad to this day that I tried my best to give Diego this natural advantage.

Seeding: how it's done
A sterile gauze is folded into a 'fan' to maximise surface area. This is then moistened with sterile water and inserted into the vagina and left to 'colonise' for one hour. The gauze is then removed and put into a sealed bag until the birth of the baby. When the baby is given to mum at birth the midwife can then pass the swab over the baby's face to mimic passage through the birth canal.

Other ways to give your baby's microbiome the best start (however they are born):
- Skin-to-skin immediately or as soon as possible after birth
- Skin-to-skin as much as possible in days after birth
- No washing of your newborn for as long as possible after birth (preferably for several days)
- Breastfeeding
- Keep baby's contact in first days of life to close family only
- Avoid antibacterial products such as soaps and washing powders
- Home birth or home surroundings as soon as possible.

associations so far, but we know that there is an association with higher risk of some diseases in babies that are born by C-section. So we need to do more research. We also have simply not studied labour enough and tried to understand what it is about labour that is healthy.'

It is in response to these early findings that some women are deciding to include 'seeding', also known as 'gauze seeding', or 'microbirthing' in their birth plans. Just like the researchers at NYU, mums – sometimes with the help and approval of their midwife or doctor, sometimes DIY – insert a sterile gauze in the vagina about an hour before caesarean birth, and then swab the baby with it in the first moments of life.

Some doctors have expressed concern about 'seeding', but it's important to stress that babies swabbed with the gauze are not being exposed to any more 'nasty germs' than they would have been had they made their way into the world via the usual vaginal route. However, if you are having a caesarean and want to consider seeding your baby, do talk to your healthcare provider. If they reel back in horror, you might like to get a second opinion, or at least remind them that neither 'vagina' nor 'bacteria' are dirty words when it comes to having a baby.

Unanswered questions

It's important to know that we really don't understand everything about the microbiome yet, not by a long shot. Here are some points to meditate on if you want to stimulate your Confusion Area.

- We know that caesarean babies have a less diverse microbiome (a). We know that caesarean babies are at higher risk of non-communicable diseases (b). However, we can't be sure that (a) = (b); we don't know for certain what role, if any, the lack of microbial diversity plays in the increased risk of disease.
- We know that washing babies should be avoided at birth and in the first few days of life to allow the microbiome to seed. But what about water birth? And is it possible to weigh up any possible detriment to the microbiome of birth in water, with the increased likelihood of vaginal birth (and probably home birth), that water birth brings?!
- And what about birth in the caul? Michel Odent believes that caul birth – when the waters don't break until baby is born – is the 'ultimate' in natural birth, and would happen to more women if birth were left truly undisturbed. Being born in the caul has long been considered auspicious, with such babies set for a long and successful

life, and many famous historical figures have been 'caul babies'. Odent asks, 'Is it not paradoxical that until now being born protected against vaginal microbes was auspicious, and that now doctors have decided to treat this as a kind of microbial deprivation?'

These questions and many others remind us of the need to proceed with an open mind, and consider just how much our knowledge of the microbiome might expand in the next few decades – or centuries! The book *The Microbiome Effect* by Toni Harman and Alex Wakeford is a great place to find more info.

Doing things the Ina May way

There is a name you may hear mentioned with great reverence among birthy-types: Ina May. ('It's pronounced Ina, like Vag-ina', she will apparently tell you.) This unassuming, twinkly-eyed American midwife has attended countless labouring women at The Farm, a commune she helped establish in the early 1970s in Tennessee. If this sounds like a hippy thing, that's because it is: The Farm was founded by a caravan of San Francisco alternative folk who believed in the holiness of life and the sacrament of marijuana. Sounds fun.

But there's something about Ina May that can't be dismissed, even by the most conventional and straight-laced obstetrician: her stats. Over a thirty-year period just over 2,000 women (from all backgrounds and circumstances) gave birth at The Farm. Of these, 94% had their babies at home or in the on-site birth centre, less than 2% had caesareans and less than 1% had instrumental deliveries. Compare this to standard rates of intervention in the US (over 30% caesarean, 5% instrumental) or UK (over 25% caesarean, 12% instrumental), and you can see that Ina May is one hippy we need to take very seriously.

To find out more about the philosophy behind these figures, I highly recommend that if you read one book in your pregnancy – apart from this one – you make it *Ina May's Guide to Childbirth*, but in the meantime, here's a potted version of some of Ina May's most well-known wisdom.

The mind-body connection

In the Western world we are used to thinking of mind and body as separate entities, but Ina May encourages us to think about what is going on, not only in our head, but in our heart and soul, and how this might be impacting on what our bodies are doing in labour. Feeling loved and adored in labour can help our cervix dilate, she says. But if something is bothering us emotionally, our labour might stall. For example, you might be worried about your partner's commitment to you with the big change that parenthood will bring, or perhaps you have a specific fear about birth that you have never addressed. Whatever it is, Ina May encourages you to clear the air and speak the words aloud; her direct experience of working with labouring women says that this usually removes any blocks and gets things moving again.

Sphincter law

According to this law, upon which all of Ina May's midwifery practice is built, your cervix and vagina are sphincter muscles and behave just like other sphincter muscles in your body (know the one I mean?).

- Sphincter muscles like privacy and familiarity (a loo door that locks, please!)
- They don't like being bossed around (commands like 'Hurry up!' or 'Push!' just don't work for sphincters).
- Just as they can open, they can also shut again if they don't feel comfortable. (Remember that time when you were just about to go but… you got interrupted?)
- Tension in the mouth, throat and jaw can prevent anal, cervical or vaginal sphincters from opening. As Ina May puts it: 'As above, so below'. Breathing, chanting, singing, sighing, moaning or blowing raspberries can all help release tension in the jaw and help sphincters open.
- The mind can have a powerful effect on sphincters. Comfort, love and reassurance can help you dilate, just as fear, interruption or anxiety can make them tighten or close.

Your body is not a lemon

Ina is a true feminist in the way she celebrates the power and brilliance of women's bodies. 'There is no other organ quite like the uterus. If men had such an organ, they would brag about it. So should we', she writes. She completely believes that women's bodies were built to birth and feed their babies, and that only a very small minority of women will struggle if they have the right support and the right circumstances. 'Remember this, for it is as true as it gets: Your body is not a lemon', she writes. 'You are not a machine. The Creator is not a careless mechanic. Human female bodies have the same potential to give birth as aardvarks, lions, rhinoceri, elephants, moose and water buffalo. Even if it has not been your habit throughout your life so far, I recommend that you learn to think positively about your body.'

Let your monkey do it

Ina May quite rightly points out that many of us have become quite distanced from the idea of ourselves as mammals, or indeed primates. She suggests that we need to let go of our analytical mind and let the older, 'monkey brain' take over. Monkeys, she points out, don't worry like we do. They don't obsess about their bodies being inadequate, contemplate how they might look in a certain birth position, do maths about how many centimetres they are dilating per hour, or worry if they make noises, fart or poop in labour. Letting go of some of this human stuff and learning to love your inner primate can help you have an easier birth.

Pain and pleasure

Ina May encourages us to think outside the cultural box. Yes, we have been taught that labour is the worst pain we'll ever experience and that we will lie on our backs on a bed, hissing at our husbands not to come near us, but does it really have to be like this, or are we falling into a trap of cultural conditioning? Can we have pain free labour? Can we smooch or masturbate through contractions? Can we have an orgasmic birth? Ina encourages us to come at labour from a different angle, and at least be open-minded about these possibilities. And if we do experience pain, she reminds us that labour pain is 'clean'; when it's over, it's over, and it almost always causes no damage to the body. The paradox is this: 'When avoidance of pain becomes the major emphasis of childbirth care... most women have to deal with the pain after their babies are born'. In other words, labour pain may be tough, but recovery from instrumental or caesarean deliveries can often be even tougher.

Hiring a birth photographer

This is a growing trend: hiring a specialised photographer to capture images, and sometimes film, of your labour and birth. Don't panic, they don't really do muff shots – they're more likely to capture dreamy soft-focus images of you looking goddess-like as you focus intently on a contraction, or glowing triumphantly as you hold your newborn. You'll need to find a photographer who has done this before and who you feel extremely comfortable with. At your birth they will stay completely in the background and use equipment that does not flash or click to distract you. Their service will usually cost several hundred pounds – but bear in mind they will need to be 'on call' for the four weeks surrounding your due date and may have to come in the middle of the night to capture your labour. And birth photographers are not just for home or vaginal births – many women who have caesareans report finding the photos extremely precious and a way of feeling more connected to their birth experience.

If you don't want to fork out for a professional birth photographer, consider if you think you will want pictures of your labour or birth and make sure you nominate someone with half a brain to take them for you. It's not the kind of life event that you can 're-stage' if you miss it!

Mother Blessings: a baby shower with a difference

Note: A mother blessing is sometimes called a blessingway, but some people object to this term because it is borrowed from the Navajo tradition and this appropriation could be offensive to them.

Ok, so it might initially set off your mung-bean alarm, but bear with me. A mother blessing, or mother rising, is quite possibly the loveliest day you will have in your pregnancy. It will elevate you to the goddess status you need to reach to become a mother, and although nobody, as far as I'm aware, has officially researched it, I have it on good authority that a mother blessing actually increases your chances of having a positive birth. Why? Read on…

Basically, a mother blessing is just a glorified baby shower, except you can lose the commercialised diaper cake and replace it with the things that money can't buy, like heart, soul, warmth and beautiful intentions. It's a chance to gather all the best women in your world around you and, as the last days of your pregnancy draw in, to really focus on two VIPs – you, and your baby.

The mother blessing party is all about you and what you want! So you can plan it to be exactly as you wish – whether you want to dance under the moon with flowers in your hair, or take six girlfriends out for an all-you-can-eat bucket of fried chicken. The main thing is your intention – it's all about celebrating you as a pregnant woman and gathering in lots of positive vibes for the amazing day of birth you are about to encounter.

Here are some mother blessing ideas you might like to incorporate. (There are lots more to be found online.) Let your imagination and creativity run wild and, just as you might with a wedding, create an event that reflects your personality and feels special and unique to you.

- Ask friends to each bring a dish of food to share to create a feast for all to enjoy.
- Ask each guest to bring a bead with them. At the party, each person strings their bead onto a thread, perhaps saying some positive words as they do so, to make a necklace or bracelet for you to wear in labour.
- Give each guest a candle to take home. When you go into labour, make sure each friend knows things are getting started so they can light the candle for you. How lovely to think of all those positive thoughts coming your way as you birth your baby!
- Make a mother blessing cake. This can be any sort of cake; the twist is that you cut a 10 centimetre round section from the centre. Why 10cm? Because that's roughly how big your cervix will dilate when you are ready to deliver your baby! You can fill this space with fresh fruit or flowers to symbolise fertility, or just to look pretty.
- Take the 10cm section of cake and give it to the men in your lives so they can have their own party. It's fun to imagine them looking at your cake in awe at the amazing tricks of the female body.
- Make a belly cast. If you have a doula she might be able to do this for you, but you can also find more information and buy kits online. Some people decorate their belly cast with paints or mosaics – another idea is to use it as a first crib for your newborn! If dads are having a pre-birth gathering too they might like to make a trestle for the cast to sit on. You can then line it with sheepskin, and know that your baby will feel very at home!
- Try henna on your bump. You can buy natural brown henna from ethnic shops or online. Ask your guests to make a beautiful pattern on your pregnant belly – depending on when you hold your mother blessing, you may still have your 'tattoo' when you are in labour! Alternatively have your bump painted by an artistic friend with a beautiful image or pattern (use non-toxic paint!).
- Bring on the pampering! Let your guests do wonderful things for you, like brushing your hair, massaging your shoulders or even giving you a much-needed pedicure.
- Make affirmations: guests write wonderful words of encouragement and inspiration for you to pin up or have nearby in labour. You could ask people to write these words on smooth pebbles you have collected, or just on circles of coloured paper which you can then string up on the wall of your birth room. You might even like the circles to be the magical 10cm diameter!

- Bring poems, songs, positive birth stories or pieces of music, and take turns to share these. If you want to get really teary-eyed, why not write and read out wishes, hopes and lovely messages to the baby, but make sure you have your tissues ready!

Michelle's Mother Blessing

I chose to have a Mother Blessing because the birth of my first child involved a heavily medicated labour and a traumatic emergency caesarean, so second time round I fully embraced all things natural, 'earthy' and positive. I hired a doula and surrounded myself with like-minded people who would help me achieve the calm, happy birth I so desperately needed.

Towards the end of my pregnancy, I gathered the women in my life at a friend's house and we made birth affirmation cards, ate cake and drank tea. We talked and laughed and each woman brought a bead to place on a birthing necklace for me. I also had a beautiful henna tattoo drawn onto my bump by a friend, which stayed on my skin up until the day labour started.

My Mother Blessing helped me get in tune with other mothers, to feel their support and encouragement. It also provided a space for me to talk about my fears and my hopes about the imminent birth and to celebrate my pregnancy journey. I truly believe that this, along with other things, really helped me achieve the healing, natural birth of my second child.

Packing your birth bag

If you're choosing to give birth in a hospital or birth centre, you'll probably want to have a bag packed and ready to go from about 37 weeks (or sooner if you are keen and organised!). If you're having a home birth, you may still want to pack a bag in case of transfer to a hospital during labour. Here are some suggestions for what you might like to put in it:

- Your birth plan and maternity notes
- A change of clothes to go home in
- Wash bag, toothbrush, toiletries, a loo roll
- Cosmetics and travel hairdryer
- Maternity pads (these are just like sanitary towels built for heavy flow), or Tena pants if you prefer
- Several pairs of comfy knickers (no need for paper pants these days, just get yourself a pack of cheap cotton granny pants)
- Nightie/pyjamas that are good for skin-to-skin and breastfeeding (easy to open at the front)
- Slippers or flip flops
- Baby clothes: vest, babygro, hat. Take three or four changes for baby.
- Newborn nappies, cotton wool or baby wipes
- Baby blanket
- Mobile and charger
- Container for placenta if needed (see page 112)
- Snacks/drinks for labour (suggestions: coconut water, Purdey's drinks, bananas, flapjack bars, glucose tablets, favourite foods to keep up energy)
- Drinks bottle or straws to make drinking during labour easier
- Supplies for partner: snacks, toothbrush, book, music, change of clothes
- One or two photos of people and places you love
- Your own pillowcase (to put on hospital pillow), or better still take your own pillow or two
- Massage oil – pure base oil with optional essential oils of your choice
- TENS machine if you're using one
- Lip balm
- Spritzer spray of water, a few drops of calming oil (e.g. lavender) optional
- Hot water bottle (can be soothing during labour)
- Birth ball if you want your own/are not sure if place of birth will supply
- Champagne plus travel cups!

If you birth away from home you will also need to remember your baby car seat to bring your newborn home.

Getting ready for a home birth

If you're planning a home birth, you may want to pack a bag in case of hospital transfer, and you'll need most of the supplies on the hospital birth bag list anyway, even if you give birth at home. But there are some extra supplies that are specific to home birth: some are practical, but you can also get ideas from the 'optional' list that will help you make a really beautiful birth space to welcome your baby.

Practical items

Floor protection. First of all, please don't panic about home birth being 'messy', as this is a bit of a myth. Your midwives will bring 'inco sheets' to protect the birth area and will be adept at clearing up without fuss, so you're unlikely to even know anyone has given birth in your house within about 30 minutes of your baby being born! To be prepared for any small spillage of amniotic fluid or post-birth lochia, or just water from the pool as you get out, you might like to buy one or two cheap shower curtains and place them on the floor around the edge of the birth pool (if you're having one), or around the bed or floor area where you think you might be likely to give birth. Then cover these up with old rugs or throws: they won't be slippery when wet and you won't feel like you're labouring in a crime scene.

Birth pool. If you have space in your house for a birth pool, get one. You don't have to use it, and you don't have to love it, but you probably will use it, and you definitely will love it. Pools can be hired, bought or you can borrow one, often via your local home birth or Positive Birth group. If you borrow one, you just need to buy your own liner. Give your partner the job of setting up, filling and maintaining the temperature in the pool. (For more info on water birth see page 157.)

Towels. Yay! You're in *Call the Midwife*! You need hot water and towels! Seriously, you'll need a few if you are having a water birth, and even if you're not, towels come in handy to wrap around you and the baby after the birth. A really nice big fluffy towel or throw, with a duvet or large blanket over the top, can cosy you both up on the floor or the sofa for some naked skin-to-skin after the birth. Any meconium (baby poo) will easily wash off, so don't worry about it and just focus on bonding.

Bucket. Some people are sick in labour. Not all. But some. You might also want to provide your own bowl or other receptacle for the placenta, depending on what you are planning on doing with it. (See page 112 for ideas).

Cake. Midwives like cake and biscuits. Who doesn't? So have plenty of tea, coffee and Mr Kipling on hand. You might enjoy a cake yourself. It's hard to know what you might want to eat in labour, so the best thing to do is to keep your options open and stock up on a selection of foods that usually appeal to you. Bananas, flapjacks, bread, energy bars, coconut water, healthy energy drinks – and anything else you think you might like. Keeping up your fluids and energy is really important.

Camera. Discuss with your partner and/or midwives beforehand what sort of images you might like. Consider hiring a birth photographer (see page 171) if good-quality film or photos are really important to you.

Mirror. Some people like to use a hand mirror to see their baby's head crowning. Yes, really.

Support person for siblings. If you have other children you need to think about who will look after them during a home birth. This needs to be someone who you don't mind having in your birth space, and preferably someone who is calm and confident, 'gets' the whole home birth thing, and who your children like! (For more on siblings at birth see page 190.)

For all other practical items, see the previous section on packing your birth bag.

Optional extras
Planning a home birth means you get to have the birth room just as you like it. With a little imagination you can turn your living room into an enchanted, twinkly and inspiring place. Here are a few ideas.

Tea-lights. Dot them round the room for a magical atmosphere. Put your partner in charge of lighting new ones when the ones that you carefully light in early labour go out. He will probably be a bit distracted by the whole labour experience and forget.

Fairy lights. Get them out of the Christmas box, or buy a string of new ones just for the big day. They will give a lovely glow, even after the tea-light extravaganza has gone out, and your partner, whom you put in charge of tea-lights, has epically failed to light new ones.

Affirmations. Think about some words or phrases that inspire you, and find some creative ways to get them up on the wall. Some people make a string of affirmations with their friends, which is an ideal activity for your Mother Blessing or baby shower. Some paint words on pebbles, or write or paint them big and stick them on the wall. Have fun with this one and be creative.

Music. Make playlists for all moods and needs. Like the food, it's hard to know what you'll fancy until labour is upon you. So put a few together, for example: music that inspires you, music with a strong rhythm (good for moving and rocking in early labour), calm and gentle tracks, nostalgic music, music that you love to dance to (can get you, and baby, moving), and, of course, songs that you imagine you would like to be playing when your baby is born. If you have your heart set on a particular piece of music for this, make sure you communicate this to your partner, doula or midwife, so that they can try and make this happen.

Essential oils. A little oil burner is a good way to bring a scent you like to your birth room. Some also like to make their own massage oil or buy a ready-blended one: rose, lavender, and citrus oils are popular for labour. Jasmine and clary sage should be avoided in pregnancy as they can stimulate the uterus, but many people enjoy them in labour. Clary sage is sometimes known as 'nature's gas and air', and a few drops on a tissue can be helpful during labour. Avoid putting oils in the birth pool though, as if you take a dislike to the scent, it is difficult to get rid of it once it's in the water. Lavender and tea tree can also be great in the postpartum bath.

Photos. Pictures of your other children, people you love, or anything else that inspires you. Did you run a marathon once? Put up a pic of yourself grinning on the finishing line. Ever climb a mountain? That's good too. Have fun thinking about times in your life when you've pushed yourself to your limits and done something amazing, and find pictures or other mementos to remind you that you thought you couldn't do it, but you did.

Rescue Remedy. My personal view is that this or any other flower essence, homeopathic remedy or herbal hocus pocus doesn't really work – and in fact, there is zero evidence to support their use. But here's a confession – I guzzled plenty of Rescue Remedy during the birth of each of my three children. Why? Because it felt reassuring, somehow. I'm not sure why. Perhaps it was just the brandy content. Whatever the reason, if you feel drawn to it, can afford it, and think it will help – go for it. As John Lennon said, "Whatever gets you through the night, is alright."

Sheela-na-gig: the ultimate birth room ornament?!

Sheela-na-gig is a rather interesting character, found carved into the stone of churches in the UK, Ireland, and central Europe. Scholars are divided about what Sheela-na-gig represents: is she a grotesque joke, does she ward off evil, or is she some kind of pagan feminine deity, perhaps (as she is often found on windows and doorways) symbolising the ultimate gateway to life?

Birth guru Ina May Gaskin thinks these figures have a message to all labouring women: you can be calm, and get big. With her calm and serene face, and huge vagina, Sheela-na-gig is here to remind us of what the female body can easily do, says Ina May:

'My idea is that this figure was probably meant to reassure young women about the capabilities of their bodies in birth. As you can see, the vulva of the crouching figure is open enough to accommodate her own head. Such a sight is quite encouraging to a woman in labor.' Ina May's Guide to Childbirth

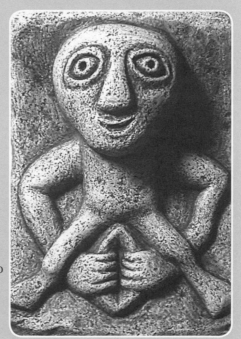

If you think that Sheela-na-gig might inspire you in labour, you can buy reproductions (statues, necklaces, paintings and more!) online, just have a google. At the very least she will ensure that any unwanted in-laws visiting after the birth won't stay too long – always a bonus.

Little touches. Dress the room just as you would for a party: birth is a special occasion. Fresh flowers, a new plant. Bunting, photos, affirmations and pictures. A little table display with some floating candles, a pretty or meaningful crystal and maybe an ornament.

The last days of pregnancy: *Zwischen*

Sometimes we just need a name for something, and our language can't provide it. What do we call those final days of pregnancy, that time when everything is ready for the baby and we are waiting, waiting, waiting? It's a tipping point, especially if we are going to become mothers for the first time. We're about to literally cross over from one state to another, and in some ways this metamorphosis has already begun: we are no longer the woman we used to be, and yet, we are not quite 'mother', not yet. Shouldn't there be a name for this?!

Zwischen: this German word means 'in between', and American midwife Jana Studelska chose to give it to these last days of pregnancy in a now well-known article for Mothering.com. Giving it a name, argues Studelska, encourages us to celebrate it as something special, rather than focusing on the inevitable discomfort and anxiety. As she puts it, the time of Zwischen is, 'an experience closer to wonder than endurance'.

It's also a time to 'dig deep'. Most of us have some time off work at this stage, and Studelska encourages us to use these days of waiting to listen to our inner voice and follow its lead: 'I tell these beautiful, round, swollen, weepy women to go with it and be okay there. Feel it, think it, don't push it away. Write it down, sing really loudly when no one else is home, go commune with nature, or crawl into your own mama's lap so she can rub your head until you feel better… I try to give them permission to follow the instinctual gravitational pulls that are at work within them, just as real and necessary as labor'.

We will need this mindset as we cross the threshold between *Zwischen* and the early stages of labour. Giving birth is not just a physical experience. Psychologically, it can help to enter a dreamlike state where you journey inside yourself, connect with your baby, and pay attention to what your body needs. It is, as Studelska puts it, a heroine's journey: 'The heroic tales of Odysseus are with us, each ordinary day. This round woman is not going into battle, but she is going to the edge of her being where every resource she has will be called on to assist in this journey'.

For some women, *Zwischen* can be tainted with great anxiety or pressure, particularly if they go past their 'due date' and begin to be asked by professionals to book dates for induction or have membrane sweeps. This special time can be entirely taken up with worry, and feelings of inadequacy that our body is already failing to work as it should. In our culture where almost everything is predictable, it can be hard to embrace the uncertainty that Zwischen brings.

I urge you to try. Just as you will never forget the day your baby is born, you will always remember your time of *Zwischen*. Try to let go of fear and pressure, and celebrate instead this chance to take a 'pregnant pause'. Gather your strength and fine tune your intuition. You will need both for labour – and for the bigger journey of motherhood that lies beyond it.

❧ chapter 8 ❧

Postive Home Birth

Why stay at home?

Deciding to have a home birth is a big leap of faith for many, in an age when most of us have been raised to see birth as a dangerous event that belongs firmly in a medical setting. Women who declare in public their intention to have a baby in their own four walls are often met with raised eyebrows and the phrase, 'Wow, that's brave!'. But of course, that's not really the case, and the evidence now is showing that, for many women, home birth may be one of the safest options. Although the reasons for this are not officially understood, I think we could all take a pretty good guess why women have better, more positive and more satisfying births with lower rates of intervention at home than in the labour ward, don't you? It doesn't take a rocket scientist to work out why a creature that performs better in a warm, cosy and familiar place where they feel safe, would perform better in a warm, cosy and familiar place where they feel safe.

Women and their partners rarely have a negative word to say about home birth. In fact, they usually speak in glowing terms, like this:

'The homebirth of my second daughter was the most amazing and empowering moment of my life so far! Being able to spend the first hour

of her life holding her while being fed cake and tea and then having a bath was just bliss. If I could give birth like that everyday I would.' Sarah Banks

'It was so much longer and harder than I expected but I felt like a warrior that I birthed a 9lb 2oz baby at home after 20 hours! I was really proud that I managed it and it was worth it for the prosecco and Deliveroo at the end – and the baby obviously!' Grace Lillywhite

'It was unquestionably the most amazing experience of my life. It wasn't painless, nor technically orgasmic, but it was ecstatic. The contractions hurt, but I wasn't suffering, or unable to cope. Birthing uninterrupted, feeling safe and supported, allowing my hormones to work exactly as they were supposed to... I entered a primal place where the pain was not bigger than me. I felt like I'd discovered the secret of the universe, and I could do it again and again.' Erin Quinn

'The thing that made the difference for me was the time after the baby was born. Being able to get into my own bed... it was just bliss.' Caroline Smith

Is home birth safe?

The best current evidence we have about 'place of birth' comes from the Birthplace study, a large-scale study completed in 2010 of over 60,000 low-risk women in the UK. The study tells us first and foremost that for healthy women with low-risk pregnancies, giving birth in the UK is actually very safe, wherever you decide to do it!

However, what's interesting – and some people find this really hard to believe – is that the Birthplace study found that for low-risk women themselves, even if this was their first baby, planning for a home or birth centre birth was safer than planning for a hospital birth in terms of avoiding major medical interventions. Caesareans, instrumental births, episiotomies, third or fourth degree tears, the need for blood transfusions and also the very rare need for admission to intensive care, happened less frequently to women who planned a birth at home or in an MLU.

If this is your first baby, the evidence says that a planned home birth is still a safer choice for you, but that it might be less safe for your baby: the chance of an 'adverse outcome' (stillbirth or serious harm) rises from 5 in 1,000 in an obstetric unit to 9 in 1,000 for babies whose mother plans to give birth at home. You're also more likely to have to transfer to hospital: around 45 per cent of first timers transfer during labour, compared to around 12 per cent of women who have had babies before.

The evidence to support the safety of out-of-hospital birth in this and one other large study is strong, and it is used by NICE in the UK in the guidelines for the NHS on choice of place of birth. If you're planning to have your baby in a different part of the world, it's important to remember that factors like geography (how far is the hospital?), and training (what training do home birth midwives have?), could mean very different statistics and outcomes. Part of what the Birthplace study shows us is that the 'belt and braces' we enjoy in the UK are part of what makes the decision to give birth at home safe. Excellent and experienced midwives who will come to your house, combined with easily accessible emergency care if you need it, is a winning combination.

If you want to have a home birth, you will need to consider your own personal circumstances and history, for example whether you have had a baby before, whether you and your baby are having a healthy pregnancy, and also look carefully at the home birth provision in your particular area, before making your choice.

Wow! You're so brave!

If you do decide to plan a home birth, you may well hear this phrase in pregnancy more times than you have to get up to pee in the night. Many people believe so strongly that hospital is the safest place to have a baby that it can be hard to convince them otherwise. We've all been brought up to believe that women would simply die in childbirth without medical interventions like instrumental birth and caesarean, but we're now coming to realise that not only do these procedures carry risks to women and babies as well as benefits, but also that some women are having these procedures when they don't actually need them. It can take time for this sort of challenging information to sink in, and people can also be resistant to it because it's so hurtful for them to think that their own birth experiences could have been very different.

In spite of the evidence, you may find that you meet huge opposition to your choices from family members or even professionals who are unable to accept the reality of the evidence we have about birth safety. Often you may be accused of being too concerned with your 'birth experience' and not focused enough on the wellbeing of your baby.

If this happens to you, gently remind your critics that this argument is too simplistic, and that in fact, everything that makes birth a more enjoyable 'experience' for the woman – homely, low-tech environments, a midwife she knows and trusts – has been shown by researchers to be optimal for safety. Remind them too, that the very fact of being in hospital can cause difficulties to the labouring woman that would not necessarily have happened had she been at home or in an MLU. And remind them that our health system provides the ultimate safety net, so that women who really do need medical help, get it.

What if I'm 'high risk'?

If you have been given the label of 'high risk', you will probably be told that home birth is not an option for you. High BMI, twins, VBAC, being past 42 weeks pregnant, or a history of health complications in previous pregnancies, are just some of the reasons that you may be encouraged to have your baby in an obstetric setting. In these cases, you need to think about your own personal condition and circumstances, as no two women or situations are the same. Women who are labelled high-risk (see page 232) can and do go on to have positive home birth experiences, while others decide that they feel more comfortable choosing a hospital setting, and of course, the final decision of where you have your baby is yours alone to make. (See page 70.)

What if something goes wrong?

There are no guarantees of everything going smoothly, wherever you choose to have your baby. However, if you are having your baby at home, it is worth noting two things:

1. Midwives are highly trained to deal with complications; they are birth experts.
2. The vast majority of complications can be spotted in plenty of time to make the journey to get medical help.

Home birth safety: professional views

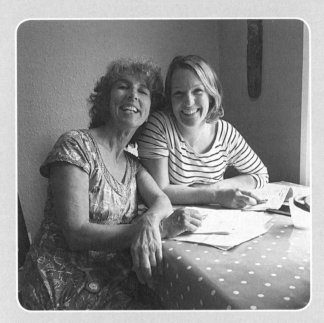

Home birth midwives Caroline Baddiley and Erika Thompson have attended hundreds of births and seen women have babies on the floor, on the sofa and even in the brand new conservatory (in a pool, of course).

We always explain to women that we are experts in 'normal' and know the paths of birth – including the twisty-turny ones – so well that we also know when it's time to seek medical help. 'Abnormal' is very clear to us.

In our experience there is usually plenty of time to arrange a transfer into hospital in a calm way, well ahead of an 'emergency', if we see signs of birth not going as well as it should.

However, if there is an emergency, we are highly trained in emergency skills and will use them immediately while also arranging for someone else to call for an ambulance. We carry drugs and equipment for emergencies and attend training regularly.

Dr Richard Porter is an obstetrician and gynaecologist at the Royal United Hospital in Bath, where the out of hospital birth rate is 20 per cent.

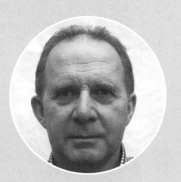

The issue of the safety of transfer to an obstetric unit in labour has been, and I suspect will always be, a tangled web. I observed over many years that the things that go wrong in the vast majority of cases (and this is particularly so with first labours), do so slowly or with plenty of warning, giving time for transfer. I recognise that the findings of the Birthplace research programme do show that delivering a first baby at home increases the risk of adverse perinatal outcome events. I confess that this result came as a surprise to me, but the figures are now there and we need to take them on board – and give mothers a balanced view of these figures. However, Birthplace also found that freestanding midwifery units are as safe as obstetric units, irrespective of whether a woman has given birth before, and that is certainly in line with what I would have expected based on more than 25 years of working closely with and supporting such units, and it runs counter to what many critics of such provision would assume – particularly as regards first labours. I still believe that the safety net is, as I have said: things go wrong slowly in most cases. The key to safe practice is remaining alert to variations from normal progress and, crucially, not taking an inappropriately rose-tinted view of them. Optimism is a necessary part of the physiological/natural view of birthing, but it should always be grounded in common sense.

What if I have to 'transfer'?

Women transfer to hospital from home in labour for a number of reasons. It's important to realise that those reasons can be complex and that it's rarely a situation involving blood, sirens and panic. Reasons include:

- Labour is taking a long time. There is no immediate risk to mum or baby's health, but she is tired, has 'had enough' or wants pain relief.
- The midwife has bureaucratic concerns about hospital guidelines or a lack of back up or second midwife.
- The midwife has concerns about the health of mother or baby. Problems can usually be spotted a long time before they become serious or life threatening.
- There is meconium (baby poo) in the waters when they break. This can sometimes be a sign that the baby is in distress, and it will be recommended that you transfer.
- Problems after the birth, such as a retained placenta or maternal blood loss, or a concern over the baby that it is felt would be best if checked.
- Serious concerns over mum or baby's health, such as a severe haemorrhage (mum) or severe breathing issues (baby). These situations are very rare but, for a truly informed choice, they must be considered when planning a home birth, just as the risks of hospital birth or caesarean must be considered when choosing those options.

If you decide to transfer to hospital in labour, you can choose to go by ambulance or by car if you prefer. If you've packed a hospital bag, take it, but don't panic if you haven't as the main focus for now is you and your baby. If you already have a midwife with you at home, she may travel with you, and will usually hand over your care when you arrive at hospital.

Deciding in labour

If you are undecided about home birth, don't worry; you can decide on the day! From a paperwork point of view, it's much easier for you to 'book a home birth', and then decide at some point in labour that you

'I felt like a warrior' – Hannah O'Sullivan tells the story of her transfer from home to hospital

I always knew that I wanted to have a home birth. I started early labour five days past my due date, and my tightenings were about five minutes apart and manageable so we spent the day pottering about the flat and going for a stroll in the park. This 'latent' labour continued for the next 24 hours and when we eventually called a midwife I was found to be 4cm. This slow progress continued, and I was tired. I alternated being in the pool and walking about to help myself dilate. I climbed a lot of stairs and was fed frozen grapes for energy! But I seemed to stick at 8cm dilated, and eventually one of my midwives suggested that we think about transferring into hospital, as it was now somewhere around 9pm on my second day of contracting.

I felt really calm about the transfer. I think this was because by now I had spent a lot of time in my own space and I really felt that my decisions were respected and that I was utterly in control of my birth. We waited a while for an ambulance as I was not an emergency, and I spent that time struggling a bit to regain my control over the contractions; in retrospect I think that was the transition phase!

I had a bag packed in case I needed to go in so that was ready and waiting. Once the ambulance arrived the paramedic crew were really kind to me. My main concern at that point was about having to travel facing backwards as I get travel sick! She helped me lie on my left side and sort of angled towards the front and the journey was super quick. I could feel fluid gushing out of me with each contraction at this point and both me and the ambulance floor were soaked! I was offered a wheelchair when I arrived but walked to the lift as I had been walking so much already I thought I might as well carry on.

When we arrived on the labour ward I was fully dilated! My midwives knew I wanted to be in the pool and so without me having to ask they went out and spoke to the team. As I was now fully dilated they suggested that I could go up to the birthing centre instead of staying on the labour ward. So off we walked again!

I really found the transfer to be a very minor part of the experience – there was nothing negative about the move at all. The way I see it is that if I had been planning a hospital birth then at some point I would have made the same journey. Having the same people around me was really reassuring and I'm sure all the extra walking around and being jiggled about in the ambulance probably helped me to progress those last couple of centimetres! In the end, I still birthed my baby in the pool as I had hoped, and I felt like a warrior!

would rather be in hospital or the MLU, than vice versa. Make sure you talk to your local midwife team in advance about this and find out what your local options are if you decide to transfer. Then just take labour one step at a time and know that your bag is packed if you want to shape up and ship out. But be warned, you might just have a baby before you make up your mind!

What about siblings?

For many, the idea of having children around at birth is pretty challenging. I remember feeling this way myself, when I planned to give birth at home with my second child, and didn't know what to do with my firstborn, who was nearly two and a half at the time. Giving this some thought forced me to really shine a spotlight on my preconceptions of birth. I realised that I didn't want my little girl to see the kind of birth I thought I would have (scary, noisy, horrific). But I was fine about her seeing the birth I went on to learn was possible (calm, peaceful, joyful). I found that having her around, dipping in and out of the room as I laboured, was absolutely inspirational, and certainly got the oxytocin flowing! I also really felt that being around such a normal, straightforward experience of birth was a real gift to her. I hope that when her own time comes to have babies, that experience will be somewhere in her memory and give her real confidence and strength.

If you want to have your other child or children around when you give birth, this is most likely to be practically possible at a home birth. However, if you are giving birth in a birth centre or hospital setting, and would like to have your other children present, speak to your care providers.

Tips for having siblings at a birth

Prepare well
Talk to your children in positive and age-appropriate terms about what birth is like and what to expect. Show them gentle and age-appropriate films of births and/or read them books or show them photographs. *Our Water Baby* and *Hello Baby* are good books for younger children (see Resources). Tell them about birth noises and make some together! Explain what mummy will be like on the day and how she might not want them to be around, or to get in the pool. Try to give them a sense of how hard mummy will be working and the ways they can help.

Enlist a special adult for them
On the day of the birth you will need someone to come and take care of them, as you may or may not want to have them in your birth space at all times, and they may well get bored and need entertaining! Try to choose someone who your children like and trust, and who can talk calmly and positively to them about birth and answer any questions they may have.

Keep them occupied
Make sure there are plenty of activities for them to do while you are in labour, perhaps making things for the baby like birthday cards or a birthday cake, or making a photo diary of the day. Once the baby has been born, they may have other important or special roles like cutting the cord, or telephoning relations with the news.

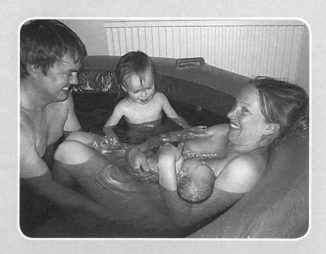

'If I hadn't been in hospital, I would have died':
the fable of the field mouse

Once upon a time there was a little field mouse. When the time came for her to have her babies, she made a nice, warm, dark and cosy nest, and began the work of every female mammal.

Now it just so happened that right at this time, a group of walkers were passing and their heavy boots dislodged the soil and grasses that were keeping the mouse's burrow hidden from view. Peering downwards at the scene, they could tell quite quickly that she was in the midst of her Mouse Labour.

'We'd better get her looked at by a professional', they decided, and scooping her up delicately in the palm of a hand, they carried her across the fields to a nearby town, and into the office of the local vet.

Once there, the mouse was taken into the surgery, and placed on the polished steel table. Bright lights were shone on her, and the vet, two nurses and one of the walkers who had brought her in, all crowded round and looked carefully to see if any mouse babies appeared to be arriving. There seemed to be no sign, so they decided to give her a bit more time to let nature take its course.

After another twenty minutes on the brightly lit table, birth still did not seem to be imminent. The vet then gave the mouse an injection of drugs to try to get her labour moving, and again they waited, watching closely for any signs of progress.

By this time the mouse seemed to be getting tired and to be in some distress. 'I don't think she's coping very well with the labour', said the vet. 'We could wait a bit longer, but my feeling is, the safest option is a caesarean'.

And so, a short time later, six little healthy mouse babies were safely delivered in the vet's operating theatre, and they, along with mum, all survived.

The party of walkers were delighted with the news. 'Thank goodness we came by at just the right moment!', they said. 'Otherwise, who knows what might have happened?!'

This is a silly story, but it has a serious point to make. So often we hear the phrase, 'If I hadn't been in hospital, I would have died!', but this statement, which often scares the be-jaysus out of anyone planning a home birth, totally ignores the effect of environment on the labouring woman, and makes the assumption that birth would have unfolded in exactly the same way regardless of the woman's location, regardless of how she was treated, regardless of how she was feeling and regardless of how she would actually have liked things to be. In other words, it assumes that the female body just doesn't work very well, and will likely go wrong, 'anytime, any place, anywhere', unless medical science is there to leap to the rescue.

I disagree. And in fact the evidence tells us it's not that simple. We know from the records of midwifery centres and private practices that, when focus is given to what labouring women really want and need, the vast majority of women, at least 80 per cent and probably more, can birth their babies without anyone so much as laying a finger on them. Conversely, we know from the records of intervention rates in childbirth that these differ widely depending on geographical area. Does this mean that women in Hull might be better built to push a baby out than those in Fife? No – it simply means that what happens to women in birth is often driven by the hospital policy and environment – and that the same woman who 'failed to progress' in the Leeds obstetric unit might have had a quick and easy time in the Cardiff MLU.

What can you do about this? Well, knowledge is power. Think about what you can do to create a birth environment in which you will have the best chance of a straightforward birth. Do your homework, make your birth plan, prep your partner, hire a doula or an IM, and choose your birth location with care. Understand the hormones of labour and think about where you personally will feel safe. And if you decide to choose home birth, don't listen to anyone who says, 'Thank God I was in the hospital or I would have died'. Because the environment you're in will affect the way you labour, whether you're a man, or a mouse.

Midwife shortages

There's an irony that occurs at the moment in UK midwifery care: women are told, 'Have a home birth!' by their midwives early in their pregnancy, and then, just as they are getting to the point where the tea-lights are purchased and the affirmations are pinned to the living room wall, they are told, 'Well, actually, you might not be able to have a home birth, because there is a shortage of midwives. If you phone up in labour, and we don't have a midwife available, you'll have to come in.'

Why it's deemed a good idea to break this news when a woman is wider than she is tall and cries when her pasta water takes too long to boil, is anybody's guess. Frankly, in late pregnancy, being told that the local shop has run out of pink balloons is enough to send you over the edge, so the last thing you need is a serious threat to the ideal birth you've pinned your hopes and dreams on.

If it happens to you, the received advice is to make sure that, when you go into labour, you have someone on hand who is able to 'advocate for you': maybe a bolshy doula or a partner who is up for standing his ground. They need to be able to absolutely insist that it is your legal right to have a midwife attend you at home, and that you are not going anywhere. 'The lady's not for turning' type stuff.

This might be needed, but far better is to anticipate this issue before it even gets raised. Talk to your care providers early in your pregnancy appointments, and tell them you have heard that this can happen. Explain that, should it happen to you, you know your rights and you still plan to birth at home. Add that you have heard that, when women really insist in these situations, a midwife is usually found, and you trust this will happen in your case. You might get known as 'that woman' (perhaps not for the first time in your life?!), but you will probably also get a midwife for your home birth, avoiding any hassle when you least need it – in your final days of pregnancy or at the start of your labour.

'Freebirth': the choice to birth unassisted

A very small group of women decide that they do not wish to be attended by a midwife in labour, and that they want to give birth at home without a professional in attendance. This might be for any number of reasons, perhaps because they have had a previous traumatic birth and lost trust, or perhaps because they feel they will birth more easily if 'left to it'. It's perfectly legal to make this choice, and it's also legal for your partner to support you in labour, as long as he or she does not take the role of 'midwife', for example by performing medical assessments. Freebirth needs careful thought, in particular if you have risk factors that may make your birth more complicated or you are a long distance from a hospital, but of course, the ultimate choice is yours.

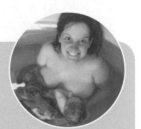

At home in the water: Beki chose to be at home in the pool for the birth of Annabel.

I was intrigued by having a home birth and after getting more information from our midwife and talking over any concerns (namely about our son George, age two, being present), my husband Graham and I decided that we couldn't wait for me to birth at home with a birth pool.

Two days after my due date, I woke up at 3am to go for a wee. I was feeling disappointed lying back in bed, as the whole of the day before I had had constant cramps, which had then disappeared. Then, drifting off, I had an unmistakable contraction, then another eight minutes later, then another…! I was so excited. Today would be the day we met our baby.

The contractions were comfortable and I lay in bed breathing them away, smiling. At 6am I woke Graham and he started getting the living room and birth pool ready while I contracted sitting up on the corner of the bed, waiting for George to wake up. Graham brought me up tea and toast and around 7am we rang the midwives to come to our house. I was managing contractions repeating a chant; 'Open. Baby'. It really kept me calm telling myself the contractions were my body opening to allow my baby to be born and remembering that meeting my baby girl was the end goal.

The midwives had both arrived by 8.30 and I was downstairs sitting at the breakfast table with my Mum, our little boy George, and Graham, who I was leaning on with each contraction. I had to really focus on my body by then, and felt immense pressure – sitting was becoming uncomfortable. After walking to the living room to have a quick examination and get in the pool, I was surprised to feel a little push at the end of a contraction. I was fully dilated, wow! Let's get in that pool!!

Graham and I got in together. I had realised then that I had no transition feelings whatsoever, which is something I was afraid of, as I felt great pain and loss of control at that stage birthing George. Anyhow the water felt fabulous, so warm, so secure, it took me in and looked after me. I was in full control and I know that being at home made all the difference. George was doing stickers with my Mum next door in the kitchen – it was perfect. After getting on my knees we got straight into pushing. I say 'we' because all the way, Graham and I felt like such a team. With only a handful of contractions and pushes, I could feel my baby's head making her way down the birth canal, it was so incredible, a fantastic feeling.

I was kneeling up with my arms over the pool grasping the midwife's arm. The water was so lovely; when I needed to position my body in order for her to be born, I could, really easily, with the brilliant buoyancy. With only another few pushes, my baby's head was born. I lay back in the water so I could feel her head and watch the rest of her being born and catch her in the water. Her body was so wriggly when she was turning, I could feel all of her, it was absolutely amazing! It actually tickled!

Finally, after what felt like forever waiting for the final contraction, our little girl swam into the world. No one touched her, I calmly picked her up and pulled her out of the water and on to my chest. Oh my goodness, the most amazing, most empowering moment of my life. I felt so high with love for our baby and great achievement. It was such a relief to finally meet her after many months of waiting. We sat altogether in the pool and George came to meet his little sister, it was a lovely family time and in amongst it our little girl was rooting and with only a little help from me, she latched on to my breast for her first feed. We got out to birth the placenta, and I reclined on the sofa with my daughter in my arms. It was bliss. Birthing at home meant my own toilet, my own comforts, not being too hot, or too cold, eating what I wanted, when I wanted. I cannot recommend it highly enough, it's the best decision I have ever made.

chapter 9

Positive Hospital Birth

Why choose hospital birth?

Around about 85 per cent of UK women give birth in hospital. The reasons for this are mainly cultural – we have all grown up being told that hospital is 'where you have a baby', and that it's the safest place, and only recently have these ideas begun to be challenged.

As you have read in the previous chapter, the evidence now tells us that, if you are a low-risk woman in a healthy pregnancy, your chances of birth interventions such as instrumental delivery and caesarean are substantially higher if you give birth in a hospital. You are much more likely to have a fulfilling and normal birth in either an MLU (see page 202), or at home (see page 182).

There may be reasons why you feel you want to, or have to, give birth in a hospital on the labour ward. For example:

- You are 'high risk' and may be more likely to need medical help at the birth
- You know that your baby may need special care when they are born
- You are sure that you want an epidural
- You don't want a home birth and there is no MLU in your area
- You are worried about transferring in labour from home or MLU
- You are going to be induced
- For your own personal and well thought through reasons, you feel safer in hospital.

If none of the above apply to you and you are still planning to give birth in hospital – I would urge you to reconsider. A home environment, or the low-tech 'home from home' environment of the MLU, will provide you with the best chance of a positive birth that proceeds without complication, and this is mainly due to the fact that you are a mammal and mammals were meant to give birth in warm, dark, quiet and cosy places.

Remember the three brains?! (see page 143). The problem with hospital birth is that your neocortex is probably a big fan, but your mammal brain remains unconvinced and your reptile brain just wants to leg it. A conversation between these three bits of your brain about hospital birth would probably go something like this:

Neocortex: Wow, I can't wait to have my baby in hospital! Look at the lovely shiny floor in here! All my friends had their babies here and I read it's the best hospital in the country on that really good website! And that doctor looks charming!

Mammalian: I don't feel safe here! There's too much space, it's all echoey, would I fit in that cupboard I wonder? And what's that beeping sound?!

Reptilian: RUN!!!!

However, if you really do have to have a hospital birth, don't despair. Armed with knowledge about the real needs of a labouring woman, you can still do a great deal to maximise your chances of a really great birth. By considering your mammalian and reptile brain's possible responses to the hospital environment, and by thinking about how these may inhibit your production of the wonder hormone of birth, oxytocin, you can make a pre-emptive strike. In other words, you can plan a 'home birth in the hospital'.

Home birth in the hospital

Hospitals are trying harder and harder to create better birth environments. However, there is still some way to go here, so if you're having a hospital birth you need to think about how you can soothe the deeper parts of your brain that may be unconvinced about the whole thing, and continue to manufacture an unlimited supply of oxytocin. Essentially you need to allow yourself to stay in your 'mammal' brain, and prevent your 'thinking' brain – the neocortex – from being stimulated as much as possible. Being asked questions, feeling that you are being watched, bright lights and disturbance, background banter and chat – all of these can draw you out of your labour trance and back into your intellectual thought processes.

Your husband or partner can play an important role in protecting your birth space, preventing your neocortex from being stimulated, and helping the oxytocin to flow. There are also practical things that you can do, even if you don't have a partner at your birth (and if you do). For more info on this see pages 128 to 131.

Kate Hewitt had her first baby in a hospital in Bristol in May 2013

We planned a hospital birth because it was that or home (there was no MLU close by), and my other half just wasn't up for the latter. He worried about something going wrong and that an emergency transfer to hospital would delay care. I had faith in my body and my ability to cope, and had no reason to think that anything untoward would happen, but expected to rely heavily on his support, wherever we were. I wondered if he'd feel more out of his depth at home, and just less safe, so therefore be less reassuring support for me. Our priority, after safety, was that it was a shared experience, for us to work through as a couple.

When we arrived on the labour ward I'd spent most of the night pacing, vomiting, trying to rest, trying to wee, swaying and stamping, swearing, faffing with the TENS machine, and, apparently, had begun to work my way through a repertoire of farmyard animal noises no one knew I had! We were shown into a room which was windowless, cluttered with clinical equipment, and bright with fluorescent lights. I was very aware of the fact that just outside the door was a very busy looking unit. I subconsciously dealt with this by retreating to the dark bathroom away from the door, and my contractions continued to ramp up, which I managed in an increasingly vocal way.

When the midwife came in I announced: 'I'm sorry about the swearing, but it helps so I'm not going to stop! I can't lie down to be examined, I need to move about a lot.' She just gave a laid-back, don't-worry-about-it half-nod-half-shrug and said 'OK, you just do what you've got to do', and turned down the lights.

We calmed and focused, settled into a rhythm. We were glad to be there and the care was just what we needed. Endlessly reassuring without being dismissive. Constantly present without being unnecessarily intrusive. The midwife owned the space, but to our advantage, offering balls, chairs, baths, heat packs, and other suggestions. All without undermining our partnership or disturbing my instinctive behaviour, both of which played an integral part and dominate my memory of the birth. She was totally unfazed by my swearing (frequent), frankness (brutal), and mess (either end), all also integral and dominant! She gently managed to monitor and ensure safety, and we were aware of team input outside the room, but not direct involvement, as we were given respectful privacy as a trio.

I stayed on my feet most of the time, leaning on the raised bed, and used the gas once I found the TENS annoying. For ages it felt like our baby was breaking through my back, which was worrying and scary. Cue more calm, unwavering reassurance, for both of us, and he was suddenly pushing down, and visible. ('I can see it, it's coming!' she said. 'No shit!' - I replied. Poor woman.) I stayed standing and our son was passed up into my arms, pink and perfect, to tears all round. He was skin-to-skin until I felt like a shower a few hours later, from which I shouted 'I could do that 100 times!'. Everyone we encountered was kind, encouraging and reassuring. We went home feeling cared for, elated and empowered as new parents by the experience.

Positive Birth Centre Birth

Why choose birth centre birth?

For many women, having their baby in a birth centre or MLU (midwife-led unit) is the ideal halfway house between the medicalised atmosphere of the hospital and the rather 'unknown territory' of birth at home. MLUs usually offer a 'home from home' atmosphere, with dimly lit rooms, comfy chairs, birth pools and sometimes even double beds where your partner can stay!

There are two kinds of MLU, known as 'alongside' or 'freestanding'. Alongside MLUs are attached to hospitals, meaning you are on the same campus or even in the same building as the obstetric unit should you need to transfer. Freestanding units are not attached to hospitals, meaning that you may face a car or ambulance journey if you need to get medical help.

If you are nervous about home birth or just don't feel your home provides the right environment – for example if you live in a shared space or in a very rural area a long way from the hospital – an MLU may well be a great choice for you. Be aware, though, that they usually only accept women who fall firmly into the 'low-risk' category, although it is always worth starting a conversation about this with your local supervisor of midwives, if you feel that you would like to birth in an MLU but have been told you do not meet the criteria.

MLUs: what does the evidence say?

Whether this is your first or subsequent baby, if you are healthy and having a low-risk pregnancy, birth in an MLU (either freestanding or alongside), is as safe for your baby as a hospital birth. It is safer for you, because you are much less likely to have interventions like instrumental births or caesarean, which carry risks.

What pain relief can I have in an MLU?

You will not be able to have an epidural in an MLU, but you will be able to have gas and air, and will usually be able to have opioids. There are often, but not always, birth pools available. You may find that your MLU midwives are interested in helping you cope in other ways, for example using aromatherapy, massage or acupressure. You may also find that the low-tech, homely environment of the MLU makes you experience labour in a more manageable way, and be less likely to need pain relief.

No room at the inn?

There can sometimes be issues with availability of space or midwives in your local MLU, and some areas don't even have an MLU. Some close at very busy times, when midwives are called to the labour ward. Find out the inside track on your local MLU by speaking to your midwives or talking to other women on social media or in your antenatal groups. If there is poor availability, make sure you let your local MP know that this issue matters to you – it might not help you, but it could help women in the future.

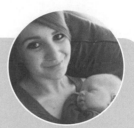

**Georgina Graham had her baby in a
London birth centre**

This was my first baby, and I was anxious,
excited, and nervous, but I also knew my mindset was
going to be important in the birth. I knew I had to keep my
environment as calm, stress free and relaxed as possible
when the time came for my baby to arrive, so choosing a
water birth and being in the birthing centre was a no-brainer
for me.

Four days past my due date, at about 8 o'clock in the
evening, I felt a tiny trickle of water and I knew this was the
start of something. Period-type pains soon started to occur,
so I called the midwives at the centre to let them know. They
were great, and told me to stay relaxed at home and come in
when my contractions got more intense and closer together
as this could go on for days. These pains very soon turned
intense and close together and by 6am, I knew I had to go in.
I arrived at the birthing centre at 7.15am and as I opened the
door I was greeted by four midwives. At that moment I felt a
huge whoosh, my waters broke! I couldn't have timed it any
better if I tried! As I had called the birthing centre on my way
in they were expecting me so the pool was already filling up.

I was taken into the room where I was delirious through
the pain I was feeling, but straight away they helped me
undress and passed me the gas and air, which was amazing!
I lowered myself into the pool and it was bliss! The warm
water instantly relaxed me and soothed the pain around my
lower back. The midwives were very calm and gave me clear
instructions and direction, as well as feeding me cool water
through a straw. The environment I was in was perfect! It
was so peaceful and relaxing, and my partner got to get in the
pool with me! In fact, I think I was so relaxed my contractions
started slowing down and the midwife told me if they slowed
down any more they would need to get me out. That was it
– I was on a mission to get this baby out! So with a few more
pushes, including a moment where I though 'I can't do this',

the head came out. I knew that this was it and that the pain would soon be over so with one final push I felt the shoulders, arms, torso, and legs slide out and was handed my baby straight away, and at 8.03am he was born. It was so magical and we just sat there in the pool for about ten minutes, staring into each other's eyes before cutting the cord.

Now I have had such an amazing experience in a birthing centre I couldn't imagine not having a water birth again! The skin-to-skin and connection we had once my baby was born was amazing, and the environment made the whole experience as stress-free as possible.

Chapter 11

Positive Caesarean Birth

Why choose caesarean?

Every woman has the right to choose a caesarean birth if she so wishes. It would be highly unusual – make that unheard of – for a woman to choose major abdominal surgery without having an extremely good reason. This might be very poor treatment and trauma in a previous birth, or a history of sexual abuse. A woman making this choice should not have to explain or justify her reasons. Asking her to do so is akin to saying, 'We just want to check if you are a total idiot or not, is that OK?'. It also probes for an explanation in a situation in which a woman would probably rather not give one, especially to a stranger.

The actual number of women who choose to have an elective caesarean is very low – around 2 per cent of all births. For the vast majority, caesarean birth is not their first choice. Regardless of your plans and desire for a normal, vaginal birth, you may find that you are going to have your baby in the operating theatre – indeed, over 25 per cent of all UK women give birth this way, in spite of recommendations from the World Health Organisation that the figure should be closer to 10 per cent. Your caesarean might be planned in advance, for health reasons like pre-eclampsia, concerns about your health or the health of your baby, or it might be decided during labour that a caesarean is the best option. If this happens, it's called an emergency caesarean, and although such cases are often not the life-or-death and urgent situation that the name implies, they can feel frightening or traumatic, and on rare occasions will take place under general anaesthetic. But whether your caesarean is 'planned' or 'emergency', it's worth knowing that there are things you can do to take ownership of the experience and make it a more positive one.

Caesareans: what are the risks?

Caesarean is major surgery. If you are thinking of actively choosing a caesarean, then it's important to consider the risks. It's also good to know the risks in case you are faced with a choice between having a caesarean or trying something different to help your baby be born, for example an instrumental birth, or just waiting a little bit longer.

Having a caesarean birth is usually very safe, but the risks include:

- A longer recovery period than vaginal birth, sometimes with reduced mobility, which some women say can interfere with caring for and feeding their baby. About 1 in 10 women say that this discomfort continues for several months.
- Infection in your scar, in the lining of your uterus or in your bladder after the operation. About 1 in 12 women get an infection after a caesarean birth, and you will be given one dose of antibiotics before surgery as a preventative measure.
- Increased risk of Deep Vein Thrombosis (DVT – blood clots). You will have to wear surgical stockings after the operation and will be advised to keep moving. You will also have a daily injection to thin the blood.
- Increased risk of blood loss, which in severe cases may need a transfusion and in rare cases (around 7 in 1,000) can result in a hysterectomy.
- Complications from anaesthetic, as with any operation. Some women (between 1 in 100 and 1 in 500) experience a severe headache, and there is a small risk of nerve damage, which usually only lasts a few weeks.
- About 1 in 10 women are admitted to intensive care after a caesarean.
- Injuries to your bladder or bowel. This happens to about 1 woman in 1,000.
- Scar tissue called adhesions can form in bands between the organs in your abdomen, which can be painful and need further surgery.
- Your baby is at higher risk of breathing difficulties due to the fluid in their lungs (this is squeezed out more efficiently in a vaginal

birth). Babies born via caesarean are more likely to have to spend some time in special care.

What do women who have caesareans really want?

We can learn so much about what is important about all birth experiences when we listen to women who have had caesareans. In many ways, the actual physical way the baby makes their exit is much less important than the way the woman feels, or is made to feel, during the birth. For a long time, caesarean birth has been quite a clinical experience, and women often report feeling very distanced from the event, as if it is something that is being done 'to them' not 'with them' or 'by them'. But all of that is changing. Women are asking for more options in caesarean, and for more recognition of the caesarean birth experience as a momentous event that they will remember all of their lives. Change is still a work in progress, but many doctors are listening to women's voices and, as a result, breaking new ground. For example, being the first person to hold your baby, or even having skin-to-skin right away after surgery, would have been out of the question a few years ago, but now more and more women are finding that they are able to have this option, and that it has a positive impact on how they feel about the birth, and their feelings of bonding with their baby. New thinking about the microbiome (see page 165) is also prompting women to consider 'seeding' their baby after caesarean birth, and many women are asking for a whole new kind of caesarean.

The 'gentle', 'slow', 'natural', 'woman-centred', or 'family-centred' caesarean

This new kind of caesarean literally puts women – and their partners – back at the centre of the birth experience, by giving them back some control and choice, and at the same time acknowledging the moment of birth as a hugely important and special time.

In a gentle caesarean, one or more of the following choices are observed:

Gentle caesarean: Jody's story

Being pregnant for the third time was a lovely surprise, although I was terribly nervous. I was nervous because my previous two pregnancies had been marred by hyperemesis gravidarum, cholestasis and the devastating news of birth defects with our second daughter. Our first birth was a forceps delivery resulting in two pelvic floor reconstructions. As a result of this our second daughter was born via a planned caesarean, which I felt disconnected from. Coupled with her health problems I now realise I was a little absent and our bonding felt strange. We were now being given a third shot at having a positive pregnancy and birth experience, so I started researching. I wanted my next caesarean to be something I would enjoy, maybe with some personalised choices. Little did I know it would become such a beautiful healing experience for us and an inspiration to others. With the help of the Positive Birth Movement Facebook page, I found a consultant who could offer a gentle caesarean, as my local hospital weren't able to help. I wanted to feel active in the delivery of my baby so needed to be able to watch the birth with the drapes lowered. I didn't want our baby to be pulled from my womb with no lung squeeze like our last caesarean – this time our baby would emerge slowly as my uterus contracted. Our baby deserved all of his blood from the placenta so we requested optimal cord clamping. I longed to be the first person to hold him so I needed him delivered straight to my chest – he stayed there for six hours. In addition to these things we also had our own music, a mirror to watch the birth and a fabulous medical team. Between them they were respectful, supportive and humorous. That day they helped to heal our hearts from previous birth trauma.

- The room is kept calm and quiet, there is no chitchat and the atmosphere is respectful
- Music of the parents' choice can be played
- The screen is lowered during the birth or immediately after so that mum and partner can watch the baby being born

- The baby is born more slowly, mimicking the way fluid is squeezed from the lungs in the process of vaginal birth
- The parents can discover the sex of the baby themselves rather than it being announced
- There is a delay in cord clamping
- The ECG dots are attached to mum's back so that she can have skin-to-skin with baby immediately
- The IV line is placed in mum's non-dominant hand so that it is easier for her to touch and caress baby
- Theatre staff stand at the birthing woman's head while the catheter is being inserted

If you want a gentle caesarean, you will usually have to discuss this with your care providers in advance, as at the moment they are not 'standard procedure'. If your care providers feel they cannot offer a gentle caesarean, you could consider travelling to a different hospital, particularly if your caesarean is planned in advance.

What about emergency caesarean?

It's really vital that you make a 'Best Possible Caesarean' (BPC) plan as part of your overall birth plan (see page 116). In this plan include your wishes for emergency caesarean, and if you want to have elements of a gentle caesarean, your care providers should be able to offer them, unless there is a very serious situation in which your health or the baby's health is compromised. It's worth talking to your midwife or supervisor of midwives in advance if you want to make sure that the hospital will be able to honour your requests on the day. If you meet with resistance, try talking to different obstetricians, as they often have different approaches, or trying a different hospital in your area. You may also like to find obstetricians who are offering wider options in emergency caesarean, and put your local obstetricians in touch with them. Your efforts might mean not only a better caesarean experience for you, but for every woman who gives birth in your local unit after you!

The MAC: 'Mother-Assisted Caesarean'

If you are interested in having a woman-centred caesarean, but want to take it a step further, you need to know about mother-assisted

Woman-centred' caesarean: Hannah's story

I'd always wanted to have natural births, but I was also very scared of this and had no frame of reference as my mother had all her babies by caesarean.

For various reasons, natural birth didn't work out for me. I had all of my babies via caesarean, but it wasn't until my third and fourth that I heard about 'natural' or 'woman-centred' c-section.

What this means is that the woman's experience is considered to be important even though she is having surgery, and those around her go to great lengths to honour the fact that she is bringing a new life into the world. What may seem like small details – the atmosphere in the room, the slower pace, the sense of reverence – all of these things give some power back to you as the birthing woman and make the experience so much more special.

In my fourth and final birth I actually had what I now learn is called a 'mother-assisted caesarean' – my surgeon allowed me to reach down with one hand and actually help him bring my baby out into the world. I could actually feel her head in the sac when I first touched her – all squishy. Then with his help I took her as she emerged. It changed the experience of birth for me – it was incredible.

caesarean, known to some as MAC. And yes, it's a big one!

In the MAC, which seems to be most common in Australia, the mother's hands – scrubbed up and gloved just like those of the professionals – are guided down to take hold of her baby as it emerges. She is then able to lift her own baby up to her chest for immediate skin-to-skin contact.

Gerri Wolfe, from New South Wales, Australia, was devastated when doctors told her that because she was expecting twins and one of them was putting pressure on a scar from a previous caesarean, she would be putting herself and her babies at risk if she went ahead with her planned vaginal birth (VBAC). By chance she came across an article about another Australian mum who had had an MAC, and to Gerri this felt like a small way of reclaiming the birth she had wanted but could not have.

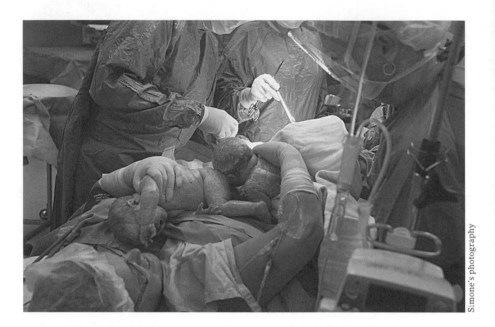

Simone's photography

Gerri negotiated her wishes with doctors at the John Hunter Hospital in Newcastle, NSW. She had already discussed with them the possibility of a woman-centred caesarean, but persuaded them to take this one step further.

'Because of the need for sterility, I had to scrub in with the doctors: soap, scrub, rinse, repeat five times. Hands up, don't touch anything. The doctor then put two sets of long surgical gloves on me and I went back to the bed for my spinal. A surgical drape was placed flat on my chest. The top set of gloves was removed. I was told quite sternly not to touch anything except the sterile drape. I had to leave my hands on my chest until told to move them. Then the doctor said, "Ok... are you ready to meet these babies?!"

'Before long the doctor had the first baby out up to her shoulders and told me to reach my hands down and feel for her. There she was – all slippery and covered in vernix. I couldn't believe it. I brought her straight to my chest.

'One minute later, I was told to reach out again. This was a bit awkward. I had my first baby in my left arm and reached out my right for my second. I had a helping hand to grab her and put her right way up on my chest with her sister. I had two slippery, vernix-covered, tiny little daughters in my arms. We just stared at them for the longest time.'

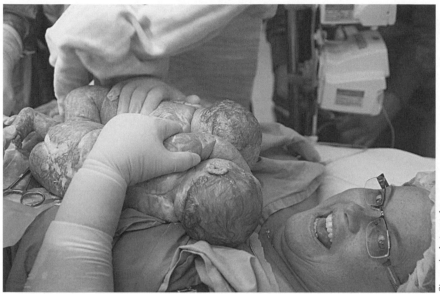

Simone's photography

Gerri's birth wishes were not without opposition: some staff were unhappy about the MAC and one theatre nurse delayed the birth by refusing to participate. Doctors are divided as to whether these concerns are valid, and if you want an MAC, you will have to speak to your individual care provider.

MAC is a new and highly unusual way of birthing. For this reason there is no research into the safety of delivering babies in this way, so if you ask for it to be part of your birth plan, be prepared to be met with baffled looks at best. As usual, it will depend very much on the mindset of the surgeon in charge as to whether your wishes are even considered: unfortunately, it's a postcode lottery.

Having an MAC is still major abdominal surgery, and it's important to be clear that it is not a glamorous or easy option. However, if a caesarean is your only option, it is a way of taking back some autonomy, as Gerri Wolfe explains:

'For me, reclaiming the birth was the whole point. Having already had two successful VBACs, I was devastated to have a caesarean and still cried for days after. But once I saw my birth pictures I realised that I did make an empowered choice. In every photo I'm smiling just like in my VBAC pics. Although it wasn't what I had planned for, it was done on my terms. I was treated with sensitivity and respect by my obstetrician and I still had an "I did it" moment.'

Woman-centred caesarean or MAC... are you allowed?!
Rebecca Schiller, of charity Birthrights, says:
'From our 2013 survey, Birthrights knows the impact that
feeling in control and respected during birth can have on
women. So, as with all aspects of maternity care, there should
be no blanket policies preventing women from accessing
these valid options. If it can be achieved in one hospital it can
be achieved in all!'

Caesarean under general anaesthetic

Around 10 per cent of caesareans happen under general anaesthetic
(GA). This can sometimes be at the mother's request, if she has
a fear of being awake during the operation, or if she is unable to
have epidural anaesthesia for health reasons. However, in other
cases, caesarean under GA can take place due to an emergency
complication, such as the epidural not working properly, or an issue
with the health of the baby. In these cases, everything can happen
very quickly and the experience can be very traumatic. Women
often feel disassociated from the birth and like they have not given
birth or do not recognise their newborn. These feelings are a normal
response to a very difficult situation. Mums who have experienced
caesarean under GA say that the following may be helpful:

- Ask for a film or a photo of the birth to be taken, in the event of a
caesarean under GA, and put this in your birth plan. Being able to
see the birth you 'missed' can help make it seem more real after
the event.
- Ask for the baby to be placed on you for skin-to-skin after the
birth even if you are not awake, or if this is not possible go for
skin-to-skin with dad. Again, put this in your birth plan and
discuss with your partner, just in case.
- Have baby for skin-to-skin as soon as possible after the operation,
and if someone experienced can help your baby latch on while you
are recovering, this can be very helpful.
- Be aware that you may feel very shocked or upset after a
caesarean under GA and that these feelings are normal and will
take time to process. Ask for a debrief to find out why your birth
happened this way and to get all of the information you need to
begin to make sense of it.

- Get longer-term support from other mums who have had the same experience via Facebook groups like General Anesthetic Caesarean Mamas Support Group, and from professional counsellors if you need it.
- Hopefully your baby will be healthy after your caesarean under GA, but please do not feel that this means you 'should feel fine'. A healthy baby is not all that matters. Your experience was tough, and you matter too.

Recovering from caesarean

Caesarean birth is still giving birth. It's really important to remember this, as sometimes, women who have had their baby via caesarean can feel like they have failed in some way or that their bodies have let them down. You might have been hoping for that empowered, 'Yes! I'm a Birth Goddess!' feeling, and sometimes, giving birth by caesarean doesn't make us feel that way. Part of recovering from caesarean may involve coming to terms with these feelings, and processing what might have been a difficult, disappointing or even traumatic experience. If you give birth by caesarean, I hope that, over time, you come to acknowledge the huge levels of courage you displayed as you brought your baby into the world, and know that you will always be able to draw on them in your life as a mother. I hope that, over time, you come to realise that you are a Birth Goddess after all. However, I'm aware that it may take a while to arrive in that place, and I would urge you to take extremely good care of yourself and get all the support you need as you make your emotional recovery.

Physical recovery after caesarean

You should be given plenty of information from your healthcare providers about your physical recovery. Here are some tips from caesarean mums themselves on getting yourself back on your feet:

'Take your time. Make sure your family know that you have been through major surgery and how tough it is, and that you will need lots of support.'

'Have plenty of skin-to-skin with your baby, not just after the birth, but in the days and weeks that follow. Focus on really bonding as part of your recovery.'

'Eat plenty of fibre and drink plenty of fluids. This will help with the constipation and gas pain that often follow caesarean surgery. Try foods rich in iron too to build your strength and lots of fruit and veg to keep healthy and fight infection.'

'I took probiotics after my caesarean. I'd read that they can be helpful to restore your gut health after the antibiotics of surgery.'

'Once the wound has healed and the scab gone away, try gentle massage of your scar to soften it. I used coconut oil.'

'Rest and sleep when you can – not always easy with a newborn! But try to make it your priority as it will help your healing.'

Breastfeeding after a caesarean

For many women, breastfeeding after a caesarean can be a very healing experience, restoring some of the confidence in your body's natural abilities that you may have lost during the birth. However, there are particular challenges to breastfeeding after caesarean, not least the fact that you have just had major surgery, which may make lifting your baby to your breast more difficult. Try to:

- Get as much help and support as you can, both during your hospital stay, and once you return home.
- Have plenty of skin-to-skin and offer baby the breast as soon as possible after the birth.
- Trust in your baby's ability to breastfeed, as well as your own. Even if you are lying flat on your back after surgery, it's possible that your baby will be able to find your breast and latch on.
- Remember that most medications are safe for breastfeeding. If you are worried, talk to your caregivers, or contact the Breastfeeding Network Drugs in Breastmilk Information Service via Facebook or on 0844 412 4665.
- You won't be able to drive for around six weeks, which could leave you isolated. Remember there is online and phone support

for breastfeeding, and plenty of peer-to-peer support via social media. (See Resources.)

- Remember the Golden Rule of Breastfeeding Success (see page 276): Scale Up. The tougher you are finding breastfeeding, the higher the level of support you need to seek.

❧ chapter 12 ❧

What if...?

'What if...?' – these are the questions that can keep us awake at night during pregnancy. This chapter aims to explore some of the situations you may find yourself in, or just be worried about finding yourself in. There are ideas about what courses of action you might take, but the emphasis is on finding the path that is right for you.

What if... I go overdue?

'Have you had that baby yet?!' People are likely to start asking you this question at around about week 36, along with helpful comparisons to 'ships in full sail', mind-bendingly insightful comments that you are 'all baby', or hilarious wisecracks about the possibilities of a twin misdiagnosis. How you will laugh.

Yes, it seems that the majority of people tend to get fixated with due dates, and actually believe that this is the day the baby will come. Babies who are born before their due date are described as 'early', and those born after it are 'late'. There is such a huge emphasis on this one particular day, that, if you are one of the many women who 'go overdue', there can be extreme anxiety, and real feelings of failure. But when research shows that less than 5 per cent of babies are born on their actual due date, is it fair for us to even think that there is such a thing as a baby being born 'on time'?

It might surprise you to know that due date calculation is based not on an ultra-modern piece of science, but on a bungled theory about moon cycles made up by a doctor called Naegele in 1812. Unfortunately Naegele didn't seem to be very good at maths, and his dodgy old sums mean that the length of pregnancy could be as much as 15 days longer than his '40 weeks' target. Nevertheless, 40 weeks remains the length of time we accept as accurate. Don't get excited about scan dates either – they are simply based on the same theory.

Research shows that the likelihood of giving birth 'on time' is exceptionally slim, and that the average first-time mother has her baby eight days 'late'. Normal pregnancy length can vary by as much as five weeks, and any time between 37 and 42 weeks can be healthy and is to be expected.

In spite of this, and the fact that due dates are pretty widely accepted to be 'only an estimate', women still find themselves coming under all sorts of pressure once they reach them, with offers of induction aplenty, and other interventions, like 'sweeps', being offered even before the due date, 'just to get things started'.

Forget due dates! Have a due month!

Why not follow the royal trend of being a bit enigmatic and telling people you are due 'in April', rather than giving a specific date? That way you will avoid the endless texts, social media messages and phone calls once you've reached your due date. Being 40 weeks pregnant is hard enough without having to field more enquiries than British Rail. Alternatively you can always refer everyone to **haveyouhadthatbabyyet.com**

So, your due date comes and goes without any action, what to do?

These can be tough times. At the moment in your life when you most need to trust in your body to work, you're being filled with doubt and anxiety and may feel like you've already fallen at the first hurdle. Take a deep breath, and don't panic.

The four main choices if you go past your due date are:

- Medical induction
- Expectant management
- Natural induction
- Do nothing

Medical induction

Medical induction for post-dates pregnancy normally takes place between 41 and 42 weeks. You will probably be offered a sweep first (see page 224), which you can accept or decline. The next step is to attend the hospital for induction. One advantage of this is that you will not be travelling in labour.

There are three typical stages to induction: prostaglandins, having your waters artificially broken (ARM), and syntocinon infusion. The aim is to do as little as possible to trigger the body to go into labour and 'take over'. So you won't necessarily need all three stages.

Once at hospital you will be offered prostaglandin gel, or a pessary, which will be inserted into your vagina, right behind the cervix. In some cases, you will be advised that you can go home after having the pessary while you wait for labour to start, and in other cases you will be advised to stay at the hospital. Wherever you wait, it may take some time, so you may wish to take books, mags, iPads and snacks to keep yourself entertained. If labour does not start after around six hours, you midwife may try to break your waters (ARM), but this is only possible if your cervix is slightly dilated. If it isn't, you may be offered another dose of the gel. If labour still does not start, you may then be offered a drip of syntocinon – but only if your waters have broken. If labour still doesn't start, you will be able to discuss the next options with your doctors.

For some people, medical induction may be the best option, but before you consent to it, it's important to realise that being induced is not the same experience as going into labour naturally. Your body and your baby go through complex processes as they get ready for labour and birth – some of which are yet to be fully understood – and a medical induction is simply not able to replicate this. If your body and your baby are ready, or nearly ready for birth, an induction might be relatively straightforward, and many women have very positive births following induction (read on for Arianwen's positive induction story). However, in other cases, induction can lead to a more difficult birth, with higher levels of pain, more need of epidurals, and increased rates of instrumental delivery and caesarean section. Being induced means that you will not be able to give birth at home, and it's very unlikely you will be able to give birth in an MLU (although it is always worth asking). The fact that your birth setting will almost certainly be the labour ward in itself makes medical intervention more likely. So medical induction is a choice that needs careful thought.

Arianwen Harris from New South Wales in Australia was induced

My baby Yazid was due on 5 December. I had managed to get a place at the birth centre. While there are a few home birth midwives that work in my area none are very close (over an hour away) and my first birth had been fast.

My birth centre midwife was lovely. I said right from the start I didn't want to talk about induction until I was at 42 weeks and that I wouldn't have any sweeps or anything like that.

My due date came and went. I felt calm although I suffered in the heat a bit. At about 40+10 I had a little wobble, but my mum and partner supported me.

At 40+11 I had a check in with an obstetrician and the baby was fine with lots of fluid. I saw my midwife around 40+12 and decided to book an induction on the day I would be 42 weeks. I asked for a sweep. On 40+13 I borrowed a hospital breast pump to try and bring labour on by stimulating my nipples, but despite a few contractions, nothing really got going.

So – in I went. As I was having an overnight induction I couldn't birth in the birth centre, but I was able to have a room with a pool. I had a pessary at 5pm and my family went home apart from my mum. We hung around and laughed at stuff. We eventually settled into the birthing room. We watched an episode of our favourite drama, *Big Love*.

At around 10ish the midwife came and gave me a second pessary. I felt deflated as the first one hadn't done anything. I was worried that this would be the start of a long induction. I talked it over with my mum and she got the midwife to reassure me.

We went to sleep but at around 2.30 I woke up and felt uncomfortable, so I walked to the midwife station to get an extra pillow. On the way back I had another contraction. When I got to the room I felt I just had to get into the shower. There were two shower heads, and I turned one on and then as I had a contraction I turned the second one on and pointed it at my belly. After a few contractions I got out and told my mum I thought things were getting going.

She thought I might be getting a bit too hot so suggested I try being on all fours in the room, but I just couldn't get comfy. After a little while she got the ward midwife. The midwife saw me have a contraction and asked to examine me. I was so desperate to be in established labour so I could use the pool.

I was 3–4 cm when she examined me so I could have the pool and gas and air. When I got in the water, it felt really great.

At some point my partner came, as did my birth centre midwife and the student midwife. The contractions were coming fast, really fast. My midwife asked me if I was pushing and I said 'I'm not sure'. My mum said, 'Yes, she is!' At one point I remember thinking, 'Where is my rest and be thankful phase?!'

The midwife asked me to get out of the pool. I said no.

She asked me again. I said no.

She asked me again and I said no.

What I needed to say was, 'I think I'll knock the baby's head if I step over the edge of the pool.'

But I couldn't. All I could say was no.

She asked again. I tried.

I moved to one knee and one foot.

Then with all my might I stood.

Out came the baby.

I looked down and made sure baby was face down as I pulled it out of the water. I noticed the cord was wrapped around the neck and carefully I put a finger under a loop and unlooped once, and then again, and as I unlooped the last half turn I saw the midwife's hands come to help. I lifted the baby to my chest and as I saw him for the first time I was struck by how much he looked like my first. I held the baby to my chest and said, 'I'll get out now.'

I felt triumphant, elated, proud.

Expectant management

Expectant management is a rather business-like term that really just means waiting a bit longer for your body to go into labour naturally, and having you and your baby's wellbeing monitored while you do so. You should be offered this as an alternative option to induction, but if you are not, you are entitled to ask for it. If you choose expectant management, you will be invited to attend the hospital, where midwives will assess your baby's heartbeat, movements and the levels of your amniotic fluid, using CTG monitors and ultrasound scans. Expectant management is something you can choose to do while you are making your decision about medical induction, not just as an alternative to it. You can review your decision making when you are overdue on a daily or even hourly basis, and expectant management may help to inform you as you do this.

Natural induction

Many people like to try natural methods of induction first before accepting medical induction, and this can often spiral into a frantic catalogue of activities, some of which have no evidence base whatsoever. It's also worth reminding ourselves at this point that just because an induction method is 'natural', that doesn't necessarily make it 'natural': you're still encouraging labour to start sooner than Mother Nature intended. However, at times when the pressure for medical induction is high, trying out natural methods can seem like the lesser of two evils. If you're 41 to 42 weeks, hormonal and determined to go for it, I'm not going to try to dissuade you. I'm too scared. So here are just a few ideas for your post-dates bucket list:

Eating several fresh pineapples. Pineapples contain bromelain, which is said to soften your cervix, although I don't know who started this rumour as there appears to be zero evidence for it. I'm also told you'd need to eat at least seven fresh pineapples to get any effect. So basically, if you want to start motherhood with a layer stripped off your gums, it's worth a try.

Raspberry leaf tea. This tea is great for drinking in late pregnancy, as it is a natural uterine tonic, and one study has shown it to shorten the second stage of labour and significantly reduce the need for forceps delivery. However, there is absolutely no evidence it brings on labour. Zero. Zilch. Diddly squat.

Clary sage. This is a powerful aromatherapy oil that has anecdotal results for softening the cervix and starting contractions. You can pour some on a handkerchief and sniff away. There have been no official, randomised controlled trials on this, so it's all hearsay, but will do you no harm. However, only start inhaling on or after your due date. Some say that even the act of deep inhalation is relaxing, which may explain its apparent efficacy.

Curry. This works on the premise that 'spicy food gives you an upset stomach' and stimulating the bowel beside the uterus can trigger contractions. This might have held true 30 or 40 years ago, when most people's idea of adventurous eating was putting HP sauce on their chips in lieu of ketchup. In modern times, however, a hot curry is unlikely to represent much of a threat to your digestive system. The most you can hope for is heartburn.

Sex. Some heavily pregnant women find this idea laughable; others are too busy shagging to even notice their due date has been and gone. It's supposed to work for two reasons: one, semen contains prostaglandin, which ripens the cervix, and two, the female orgasm produces oxytocin, an essential hormone for labour and birth, and the associated uterine contractions have been known to kick-start the birth process. If you feel like it, do it – unless you've been advised to avoid it for medical reasons.

Castor oil. This stuff has a flavour like melted tea-lights, and it certainly has a most dramatic effect that could potentially save you a lot of money on colonic irrigation. Because of this, ahem, explosive action, it does actually – I'm told – work for some people. If you want to try it, have a good night's sleep and start the day with a tablespoon mixed into food or fruit juice. Then stand back and wait for the fireworks to begin. Stock up on loo paper first.

Membrane sweeps. This involves a midwife 'sweeping' her finger around your cervix and separating the membranes of the amniotic sac from the cervix, which is said to release prostaglandin hormones and trigger labour. These seem pretty homespun and friendly; no sinister drugs – just a midwife and her finger, and many of us accept them without question. Do they work? How could we ever really know? Most women who have them are due to start labouring any day, so anyone who does begin after being 'swept' surely can't be sure that it was this that actually got things moving. Or perhaps there's a placebo effect – they work if we think they will. If you want to try a sweep, remember they aren't without risk – your midwife may accidentally rupture your membranes, meaning you will be up against the clock to labour spontaneously and thus may face medical induction anyway. Remember, a midwife should not give you a sweep, or break your waters, without your express permission. If you are having an internal examination of any kind and want the professional involved to stop, insist that they do so.

There's a longer list, of course – acupuncture, reflexology, nipple stimulation and evening primrose oil pessaries are just a few more choice activities you can indulge in as you lumber around with a full-size baby trapped in your innards. I understand your sense of desperation, but I do want to assure you of one key fact: you are going to have a baby, and soon.

It's important that the stress that this desperation inevitably brings doesn't backfire on you, making it hard for you to relax and get in your zone, and ironically delaying the process you're so keen to get started. Rather than a pineapple and castor oil mocktail, it might be fruitful to ask yourself if there are any mental or emotional blocks that are holding you back from labour. (See page 142.) Perhaps even have a glass of wine instead, and a long and honest conversation with your partner about your hopes and fears, followed by a cry and maybe some lovemaking. That's got a good chance of working.

Alternatively you could try my patented method, which I'm hoping will make me unfeasibly rich:

Do nothing

Yes. You heard me. Do absolutely nothing. Don't google anything. Don't swallow anything. Don't run up stairs sideways. Don't do anything. Just believe you will go into labour soon. Breathe out. And wait.

Doing nothing. It takes a cool resolve, a mindfulness, and a deep and strong belief in yourself and your baby and your body's ability to work. Exactly the mindset you need when you go into labour, funnily enough. Don't let your confidence be undermined. Just believe. Breathe. Wait. And do nothing. Try it. It's harder than you think.

Of course, you don't have to just 'do nothing'. You don't have to just 'accept induction'. The time when you are overdue stretches out in a large lazy yawn, as if mocking your stubborn cervix, which refuses to do the same but instead stays clamped tightly shut. So in this hinterland, this time of 'Zwischen' (see page 180), you will have space to try as many options as you wish. On Wednesday morning you may decide to try my patented Doing Nothing method. By about 4.30pm you may find yourself wondering if a Piña Colada might be acceptable and effective, so long as you add a couple of tablespoons of castor oil. Twenty-four hours later you may be keen to hand yourself over to the obstetricians, or indeed, to anyone in authority who will have you and more importantly get the blimmin' baby out by any means necessary. I do know what it's like. I've been there. Take your time, and do what you need to do.

As you explore your options, here are a few more points to consider:

- How 'overdue' actually are you? Remember that 'normal gestation' is considered to be 37 to 42 weeks. Many leading bodies, including the World Health Organisation, define a prolonged pregnancy as being past 42 weeks, and yet many women are induced at around 41 weeks, or even before.
- The evidence that we have seems to point to a very small increased risk to the baby as the pregnancy goes further post-dates. You may be told that 'your risk of stillbirth doubles' after 42 weeks, and actually, according to much of the evidence, this is true! But putting it in these terms, known as 'relative risk' (comparing one risk to the other), makes the risk of stillbirth sound scarily high. In fact, most of the evidence tells us that the 'absolute risk' (what the risk actually is, not how it compares to other risks) of stillbirth in week 41 is around 1 in 1,000, in week 42 it is around 1.5 in 1,000, and in week 43, around 2 in 1,000. The risk of stillbirth is very low, and increases slightly as your pregnancy goes further post-dates. There are also many other factors that increase your risk of stillbirth, such as smoking in pregnancy, very high BMI, and low socio-economic status, which cannot necessarily be separated out from going past your due date.
- Is there a history of longer pregnancies in your family, or have your previous pregnancies been long? Evidence shows that genetics has a very strong influence on your length of gestation. If your mum had you at 42 weeks, you might be in for a longer wait.
- What kind of birth have you been hoping for? If you want a managed birth in hospital with an epidural, then getting induced

might not be such a big deal for you than if you have been hoping for a natural birth or a home birth. Likewise, if you want to birth at home or in an MLU, you might find some resistance to your plans if you go past 42 weeks pregnant. (See 'What if... I'm told I'm not allowed' on page 251.)

- If you decide to have a sweep (see page 224), or even if you don't, you can ask your midwife to tell you how 'favourable' your cervix is. She will be able to examine you and assess your cervix – the position it is in, how soft it feels, how thin it feels, and whether you are at all dilated. This is sometimes called assessing your 'Bishop's Score' (just when you thought there was one part of your body left that would never get a rating). It's important to remember, though, that even if you get a really crap score, your cervix can suddenly spring into action and win all the prizes. You might also like to think about assessing your own cervix – if you want to, you can read more about the Bishop's Score online and then make your own judgement of your own progress.
- There might be talk of big babies if you go past your due date and you will certainly feel that you are getting unfeasibly enormous. For more on big babies, see page 252.

And finally...

Sometimes the situation of being overdue can really put women into battle with their care providers. Often the most sensitive language is not used; for example, you might be told, 'We are booking you in for induction next week', and you might not feel that you are being given a full picture of your choices or having the evidence properly explained to you. This can cause some women to withdraw from their care providers entirely, and, while this is still a choice that you are free to make, it is not necessarily the best or safest one. In a more ideal situation, women and care providers would work together in a mutually respectful alliance, each realising that they have experience and wisdom to offer the other. If you can, try to work towards this dynamic in your own care. Try to stay in a positive relationship with the professionals caring for you and your baby if you can, and if you do not feel happy with the advice and support you are being given, remember that you can ask to speak to a more senior midwife, the head of the unit, or the supervisor of midwives. Above all, keep connected to your own body and your baby, remaining flexible about the many ways that your forthcoming birth may unfold.

What if... my waters break but my labour doesn't start?

In spite of what the world of soap opera would have us believe, most women's 'waters' – the bag of amniotic fluid that surrounds the baby – don't break until near the end of labour. Some don't break at all, and the baby is born still in its sac, or 'in the caul', considered a portent of a long and successful life. But for around 10 per cent of women, waters break before labour starts, and although in most cases labour will get going within the next 48 hours, for some, it doesn't.

In other cases, waters are broken accidentally during vaginal exams or membrane sweeps. Whether your waters were broken by an over-enthusiastic midwife, or spontaneously, the problem you now face is the same – if your labour doesn't get going soon, you might find you are under pressure to be medically induced.

Obviously, if your waters break or you notice any leaking before 37 weeks (known as Preterm Premature Rupture of Membranes, or PPROM), you need to seek the advice of your care provider immediately. PPROM may mean that you are going to go into labour early, and there is also, as with Premature Rupture of Membranes (PROM), a risk of infection. You can find more information and links about PPROM in the Resources.

However, if you have reached 'term' and your waters break, you may receive differing advice depending on the area of the country or the part of the world you are living in. Some women are advised to be induced immediately (and if you have Group B Strep, there is evidence to support this). Others are advised to be induced if labour does not start after 24 hours, while others are told they can wait longer: 48 hours, 72 hours or even 92 hours before medical induction. Some are told to attend for induction urgently, only to find on arrival that they have to wait as no beds are available. Some are given antibiotics, others are not. Amid this medley of options, it can be hard to know which is the best and safest path.

As with all birth choices, a good place to turn for clarity is the NICE guidelines (see page 151). In this case they currently advise that you are offered a choice between expectant management (waiting and being monitored), and induction, and that induction is appropriate 'approximately 24 hours after PROM'.

The reason for the concern over PROM is that, once the membrane sac around the baby is ruptured, the risk of infection is increased. This is because infection can more easily reach your uterus and your baby.

Researchers have looked into what is the best choice for you to make if your waters have broken, but labour has not started yet. The biggest piece of research is called the TermPROM study, and it happened in 1996. This study did find that the chances of infection were higher in the mothers who waited up to four days, versus those who were induced (8.6 per cent and 4 per cent respectively). However, this and other studies that have found an increased risk in waiting did not take into account the number of vaginal exams (VEs) the woman had while she waited.

Vaginal exams can introduce infection, not from the clean, gloved hand that gives them, but from the woman's own vaginal bacteria which is pushed further up towards her cervix when she is examined. Several different studies have found that your risk of infection after PROM increases with every vaginal exam you have. Therefore it's important, regardless of whether you decide to be induced or wait, that you keep VEs to a minimum, or have none at all.

Overall, the research seems to say that the risk of infection after PROM is low and that both being induced and waiting are valid options with their own advantages and disadvantages.

If you choose to wait and be monitored, remember:

- Take your temperature every four hours as this can be the first sign of infection.
- Limit VEs as much as possible.
- Do not have sexual intercourse, as this can also introduce infection.
- Use a clean pad for your leaking waters and do not use tampons.
- Rest, eat and drink and take care of yourself.
- Bath and shower as usual.

Report immediately any changes such as a rise in temperature, feeling unwell, hot, shivery or sweaty, change in the colour of your waters, reduced baby movements, bleeding, or pain.

What if... I tear or am cut during birth?

This is another huge fear that women have before labour and a delightfully gory feature of many a birth horror story. It's hard to imagine that arguably the most delicate and intimate part of your body could be damaged in this way, and even thinking about it is sure to make you wince. Then you'll hear stats like '90 per cent of women tear in childbirth'!!! And bingo, you're terrified.

And now you want me to tell you that the 90 per cent stat is not true, right?! Unfortunately, I can't. Because it is.

But don't panic. First of all, women often report that the sensations of crowning and the head being born (see page 37) are so powerful and intense that they don't actually notice that they have torn until they are told about it afterwards. Most perineal injuries will be small, and some will not need to be stitched but will heal perfectly well by themselves, just like any other minor cut or graze on your body. These tears are known as '1st and 2nd degree'. First-degree tears will not need stitches. Second-degree tears will usually be stitched, but some argue it's better to leave things to heal naturally if possible, as stitching introduces more trauma to the area. Check with your midwife and if she thinks it's possible to skip the stitches, do.

More serious tears are called 3rd or 4th degree and these are rare, happening in only around 5 per cent of cases for first-time mothers, and in 2 per cent of women who have had a previous vaginal birth. They will need stitching and will be more uncomfortable after the birth and take longer to heal than 1st and 2nd degree tears.

Episiotomy

In some cases your doctor or midwife will perform an episiotomy. This is a cut to the perineum and is done to help your baby be born, for example if they are in a difficult position, or if they need to be got out quickly, or if an instrumental delivery is suggested. You will be given a local anaesthetic or an epidural. After the birth, you will have stitches and you should follow the instructions given to you by your care providers to look after your perineum and promote healing.

Looking after your perineum: before, during and after birth

You might not have paid your perineum much attention before this point in your life; in fact, even the word might be new to you! It's a somewhat overlooked part of our anatomy, but when it comes to pregnancy and birth, it's important and must no longer be neglected.

Before the birth. Some women prepare by regularly massaging the perineum during pregnancy, from about week 34 onwards. Research has suggested this may improve elasticity and prevent tearing, and you can find step-by-step instructions if you google 'perineum massage'. Some women feel this is a positive action they can take, and others even purchase a gadget that will do the job for them, called an Epi-No. ('Epi? No thanks!', you may say, but one midwife I spoke to swears they make 'first time perineums act like they've had babies before'). 'Kegels', or pelvic-floor exercises, are also suggested by some to tone the area in pregnancy, but others argue that you don't want taut muscles in this area during birth – quite the opposite – and that these are best left until after the baby is born.

Will all of these frantic, and frankly rather oily, workouts simply make us obsessed with 'fixing' or 'improving' this 'problem area', bringing yet more fear and negative thinking? Or could this massage be a positive or sensual experience that makes you feel less inhibited and more familiar with this part of your body? Only you can decide, but if you want to get the coconut oil out – go for it.

During labour. Now here you really can help your perineum. Active upright birth will reduce your risk of tearing or needing instrumental delivery, as will water birth. If you are not birthing in water, a very warm flannel applied to the perineum during crowning has been shown by researchers to reduce tearing and pain. Also avoid being told to 'push' when you are not ready, or encouraged to push really hard, as this so-called 'purple pushing' is more likely to result in tearing. Listening to your body and letting everything stretch slowly is a much better plan.

After birth. Now is the time for gentle pelvic floor exercises, which may feel impossible at first, but will soon bring improved tone and sensation. Keeping any grazes, tears or stitches clean with a quick twice-daily bath in warm water with perhaps salt, lavender or tea tree oil added is a great idea and very soothing. If you experience stinging when you wee, try pouring a jug of water over the sore area while you urinate. Using ice packs wrapped in a soft cloth can help a particularly sore perineum, and some add a mixture of diluted witch hazel, essential oils and soothing herbal tea such as chamomile or comfrey to postnatal pads and then place them in the freezer before use. All women, regardless of whether or not they have had stitches, feel anxious about their first poo after having a baby. Drinking plenty of water and eating healthily can help prevent constipation. You will survive it!

What if... I'm 'high risk'?

'High risk' is a catch-all label that is applied to any woman who doesn't fall into the 'low risk' category during pregnancy and birth. Arguably, neither of these labels are particularly useful, since they not only encourage a 'one size fits all' mentality, but they also, once again, ensure that we think of birth in terms of risk and danger. Even women who have perfectly straightforward and healthy pregnancies are still categorised in terms of their level of 'risk'. Hey girl, you might be in the prime of your life and your body might be doing something pretty flippin' awesome, but we're going to call that state 'low risk' anyway. Hmmm.

You can see how the labels might be well-meant, and useful to those who have to fill in forms and tick boxes on a daily basis. However, if you're one of the 55 per cent of women who are given the high-risk label, it can make you feel rather doomed, and unfortunately, it can also make you feel like your birth choices are more limited than those carefree 'low riskers'.

You may be declared high risk for quite a large number of reasons. Some are fairly clear-cut; for example, you may have an underlying health condition like heart disease or cancer, it might be discovered that there is a health issue with your unborn baby, or you might develop a pregnancy-related condition such as pre-eclampsia, which poses a threat to you or your baby's wellbeing. In these situations, 'high risk' is not likely to be a label you would take any issue with, and you will almost certainly be happy to have your pregnancy and birth monitored and managed by doctors, who have high levels of expertise when it comes to the body not working as it should.

However, there are high risk 'grey areas', and falling into them can be frustrating and restrictive. For example, if you have a high BMI (Body Mass Index), you will probably be told you are 'high risk'. This may mean that you are told you may not have a home birth, or use the birth centre, and that hospital birth is your only option. You might also be told that you cannot have a water birth in any setting. However, this advice might vary depending on geography. Some birth centres might accept you if you have a BMI of 35 or under, while for others the cut-off point may be 40. Some may take other factors into consideration, like your personal history and overall health, while others may be more unyielding.

Similarly, if you are an 'older mum' (there's another lovely label!), you might be told you are high risk and that you need to have your baby in hospital or even be induced early. Likewise if you are pregnant with twins, even if they were conceived naturally, you may be told that your birth needs to be medically managed or that you will need to have your labour induced. However, women in other areas of the country or the world may get different recommendations in the same or similar situation.

In all of these examples – high BMI, being older, or carrying twins – you may feel that you are perfectly healthy. It's important that your situation is assessed on a case-by-case basis, and that you are treated as an individual and not a diagnosis. For example, a woman having her second baby at 41 who is in great health and had a spontaneous vaginal birth with her first, cannot be compared to a first-time mum of the same age who has a high BMI, a poor diet and is a smoker. It's also important that you are encouraged to make informed choices about your care and never told that you are 'not allowed' to take your chosen path. (See pages 70 and 251.)

Women who are 'high risk' do still make the choice to birth at home and some negotiate a place in a birth centre. Some feel that it's arguably even more important for high-risk women to be in an environment that puts them at the lowest risk of complications. If you are high risk, it's best to talk to your care providers about the kind of birth you want, and also to talk to other women who have been in your situation and find out about the choices they made (see Resources). Some high-risk women find an independent midwife very helpful, or a doula who has experience of their particular risk factor or situation.

What if... I have gestational diabetes?

Gestational diabetes (GD), a type of diabetes that appears in pregnancy and disappears again after the baby is born, is on the rise. There is speculation that this could be because of rising BMI levels, and the overall tendency towards obesity and high-sugar diets. Whatever the reason, around 6 to 8 per cent of women will be diagnosed with GD in pregnancy, which basically means their blood sugar is abnormally high.

You can reduce your risk of developing GD by adopting a healthy lifestyle before pregnancy and making sure your BMI is below 30. You can google 'BMI calculator' to find out your BMI if you don't already know it.

My high-risk birth: Erika Townend

It was a smooth pregnancy with exciting times ahead – a house move to a new area and a baby shortly after. Towards the 28th week of the pregnancy I had a midwife appointment with the usual urine test, which unfortunately flagged up 'sugars'. I had no idea what this all meant, but just listened to the advice of what would happen next. I was referred on for a Glucose Tolerance Test (GTT), which showed that I had borderline Gestational Diabetes (GD). I was told that it could be treated via diet.

Every Monday became the laborious GD clinic, where irrespective of your appointment time you could guarantee an afternoon of Woman's Own magazine reading! Fast-forward to around week 36; my blood sugar readings started to increase and insulin injections were recommended twice a day. During this time I was attending NCT classes and fortunately our teacher briefly talked about having choices. This was pivotal to how our birth unfolded.

Under NICE guidelines at the time someone in my situation would normally be induced at 37/38 weeks, but the idea of being induced so early on felt wrong to me on every single level. I wasn't scared, but I felt healthy and was enjoying my pregnancy. On the following Monday I expressed my wish to be induced later on or after my due date. Viewing my history they had no problem, and in fact they didn't even flinch at the idea. We waited until I was 40 weeks pregnant and following having my waters broken and a little help with syntometrine, my beautiful baby boy finally lay on my chest as I chanted, 'I have a baby... I have a baby...' in total disbelief. At no point did I doubt that I would birth my baby, and I was beautifully supported by my husband and my best friend.

If you have a history of diabetes in your family, have had GD in previous pregnancies, have had a previous baby over 4.5kg (10lb), have a BMI of over 30, or have South Asian, Chinese, African-Caribbean or Middle Eastern family origins, you will be considered at higher risk of GD and offered a screening test, called the Glucose Tolerance Test (GTT), in pregnancy to see if you have it. The GTT involves a blood test taken before, and again two hours after, a drink containing a high level of glucose.

If you don't have the test (either because you decline, or because you are not considered at risk and are therefore not offered it), it's unlikely you will know that you have GD, as it does not usually have any symptoms. GD may not cause you any problems in pregnancy, but it does increase your risk of having a larger baby, which in turn increases the risk of shoulder dystocia. GD can also cause problems like newborn jaundice, premature birth, and pre-eclampsia.

Some are critical of the whole concept of GD, saying that it is just another way of 'pathologising' pregnant women. Some question the accuracy of the test, and obstetrician Michel Odent calls GD, 'a diagnosis in search of a disease', suggesting that the advice given to women who have it – to exercise more and eat a 'low GI' diet (fewer fizzy drinks, more fruit and veg, fewer potatoes, more wholegrains), should simply be given to all pregnant women. Certainly many women who get a GD diagnosis find it has a negative effect on their pregnancy: they report feelings of guilt and worry about their baby, along with feeling a loss of control and sense of restriction by the many new rules given to them by care providers.

The best course of action, regardless of whether you have GD, are at risk of GD, or have no issue with GD at all, is to exercise or be active, and eat a healthy, balanced diet during pregnancy, or before you even get pregnant if you can! Choose foods that are low GI (google for lots of menu ideas), and avoid high-sugar foods like fizzy drinks and sweets. Some suggest that taking this proactive approach might even reduce your chances of a GD diagnosis, and there is certainly no harm in trying!

If you do get a GD diagnosis, diet and exercise will be the first suggestions to help you control your blood sugar levels. If this is not effective, you may be offered tablets or insulin injections. As always, you may wish to ask questions of your care providers and the BRAIN acronym (see page 119) may be especially useful to you.

What if... I have a high BMI?

Being overweight or obese is defined as having a BMI over 30. Around 15 to 20 per cent of UK pregnant women now fall into this category, and this figure is higher in some other parts of the world, such as the USA. If you're already pregnant, you will probably find that your BMI is calculated at your first midwife appointment, and if it is found to be over 30, you will be informed that you are at increased risk of complications such as gestational diabetes and pre-eclampsia, and difficulties at the birth such as problems siting an epidural, and an increased likelihood of instrumental birth and caesarean. This may affect the type of care and the birth options that are offered to you (see What if...I am high risk? on page 232).

If you are told you have a high BMI, ask to see the policy of the hospital you plan to give birth in, and, if you want to negotiate birth at home or in a birth centre, speak to your supervisor of midwives. It's useful, too, to speak to other mums with high BMI about the options they were offered and the choices they made, via your social network or groups like Big Birthas (see Resources).

What if... I want a VBAC?

VBAC – pronounced 'veebac' – stands for Vaginal Birth After Caesarean. In other words, if you have had a previous baby via caesarean section, but have the next one vaginally, this is a VBAC. If you have had more than one caesarean this is known as a VBA2C, VBA3C and so on, and if you have a Home Birth After Caesarean, this is known as, yes, you guessed it, an HBAC.

VBAC is a hot topic when it comes to the so-called 'politics' of childbirth. This is because in some parts of the world care providers will simply not allow a woman to VBAC – it's banned, for example, in around 40 per cent of American hospitals. Some UK women also meet huge resistance if they state that they want a VBAC, often being labelled 'high risk', while others report that it is simply assumed that they will birth vaginally, and still others meet resistance to requests for a repeat caesarean.

The reason for some health professionals' concern over VBAC is that, once the uterus has been cut into during a caesarean, the scar tissue this leaves is said to be at higher risk of rupture during a subsequent labour. If your uterus ruptures during labour – and this can happen to women who have not had a previous caesarean too – it is a serious medical situation requiring an immediate caesarean.

Women wanting a VBAC will be told about the risks of rupture and it can certainly sound scary. However, some feel that these risks are framed in a way that deters women from VBAC, or are overstated in comparison to other risks associated with all birth.

How VBAC risks are framed

The most-quoted figure for the risk of uterine rupture at VBAC is '1 in 200'. We do not have extensive evidence about VBAC, so it must be stressed that this figure is not specific to individual women; it does not take into account, for example, their health, age, mindset, medical history, number of previous caesareans, how long ago those caesareans took place, what kind of incision they had, whether their labour was induced (which increases rupture risk) or any other number of factors. However, even if we accept this figure as an accurate representation of the risk, it's interesting to consider the other ways it could be stated. For example, '1 in 200 will rupture', could also be framed as, '50 out of 10,000 will rupture', or indeed, '9,950 out of 10,000 will not rupture'. Likewise 'the risk of rupture is 0.5 per cent' could also be stated as, '99.5 per cent of women do not rupture'.

How VBAC risks are overstated

Most women who plan a VBAC will be told, often fairly extensively and by several different healthcare professionals, about rupture risk. However, women are told less often or not at all about other risks of birth with similar stats. For example, the risk of cord prolapse in any birth is around 0.5 per cent, and the risk of shoulder dystocia in any birth is around 0.7 per cent – and both of these are considered an emergency situation. But how many pregnant women are given this information?

VBAC versus repeat caesarean

Women who have had one or more caesareans have a choice to make between VBAC and another caesarean. Leading bodies such as RCOG, ACOG and RCM support both choices. While VBAC carries the small risk of rupture, caesarean birth also carries risks, and these risks grow each time the surgery is repeated. For example, the more caesareans you have, the more likely you are to develop adhesions, bands of internal scar tissue that can be painful.

What about HBAC?

Some women choose to have a home birth after caesarean, often because they feel that the calm and familiar surroundings of home give them the best chance of a vaginal birth. In the rare event of uterine rupture, your baby will need to be delivered within 30 minutes, so you may like to think about your distance from the hospital. The risk of uterine rupture is lowered with every successful VBAC a woman has, and this prompts some to have their first VBAC in a hospital setting, then subsequent VBACs at home. As with all other birth choices, it is up to each individual to consider their own risk factors.

What are my chances of 'successful' VBAC?

It's terrible to talk about birth in terms of success or failure, but unfortunately a lot of the language around VBAC uses these sorts of words. In the UK the chances of a vaginal birth in a planned VBAC are around 2 out of 3, but this varies depending on the type of care you receive, and where you have your baby. You can find your local hospital's VBAC rates on the Which? Birth Choice website (see Resources), and you may also like to ask your local independent midwife for her VBAC rates.

Support for women wanting a VBAC

VBAC can be very confusing territory for women, full of mixed messages and seemingly contradictory statistics. Added to this, many women who are considering a VBAC have had a previous difficult birth and both they and their partner may be feeling added layers of worry about this subsequent experience. You may wish to consider hiring a doula or IM, or talking to other women about their experiences and decisions. You can find suggestions for VBAC support in the Resources.

What if... my baby is born prematurely?

'Try to feel how it is if you are a mother, standing outside an incubator, your precious child suffers and has a very tough way of living.' These are the words of Dr Uwe Ewald, Professor of Neonatology and Director of the Neonatal Intensive Care Unit (NICU) in Uppsala, Sweden. His capacity for empathy seems extensive. Looking back on his long career in the NICU, he reflects on the 1970s, when survival rates in premature babies rose due to new technology, but in his view, not without drawbacks:

'At that time we didn't recognise that small babies were living humans with emotions and pain', says Dr Ewald. 'We couldn't see that they struggled and were suffering.'

In allowing himself to see things, not just from the perspective of parents, but also of the premature babies themselves, Dr Ewald seems to be a pioneer. For the most part, it is accepted without question in the NICU that the baby will be separated from their mother and father by being placed in an incubator, but Dr Ewald is one of a number of professionals leading a trend that acknowledges the importance of parents being much more included in the care of 'preemies', and of skin-to-skin contact. This benefits not just the baby, but the parents too, who often report feeling surplus to requirements in the NICU or the Special Care Baby Unit (SCBU).

The unit in Uppsala is unusual in that it is set up so that parents can be there 24/7, not sitting in chairs beside the incubator, but more often in a bed, with their baby held skin-to-skin on their chest. Parents are also given training in how to use slings, so that they can move around the unit, with their baby held close and attached to small mobile monitors in their pocket. However, in most cases, says Dr Ewald, the parent will detect problems with their baby several seconds before the monitor.

Kangaroo care

This kind of care for premature babies is called 'kangaroo care'. Kangaroo care, where the baby is held in close skin-to-skin contact for as much of the time as is practically possible and appropriate to their level of need, has been shown by research to reduce mortality, and it has huge emotional benefits. Babies are not separated from their parents, meaning that attachment and bonding can take place. Parents feel empowered and involved in their baby's care. Breastfeeding is promoted, and stress levels in both parent and baby are reduced. In follow-up studies, parents who have been able to give kangaroo care to their premature babies have been shown to feel less shame and guilt about their NICU/SCBU experience, and have fewer depressive symptoms than those parents who were not able to care for their babies in this way.

This kind of thinking has been slow to take root in healthcare systems despite the evidence, but is very much worth knowing about if your baby is born prematurely. Even if your NICU or SCBU is not set up for this kind of care, it is good to know that it is taking place elsewhere in the world, and so, if you want to be more involved in the care of your premature baby, practise kangaroo care, or just simply hold them, you have the right to ask for this – they are your baby! It's completely normal to want to hold them in your arms; indeed, you are hardwired to want and need this deeply, just as they are hardwired to want and need to be held by you. If you meet barriers or feel your access to your baby is not as good as you would like, seek support (see Resources). And don't be afraid to tell staff exactly how you feel – your feedback may pave the way for positive future change.

Breastfeeding your premature baby

Breastfeeding provides a number of long-term benefits for all mothers and babies, and is even more important for premature babies. However, due to mother and baby separation (some of which is unavoidable with a preemie, some of which, as discussed, could be improved upon), there are challenges to initiating and maintaining lactation in the NICU. Good help and support is therefore even more important for you and your baby. If your baby is strong enough to suckle, it is advisable to put them to the breast as soon as possible. If they are not yet strong enough, you should start to express as soon as you can after the birth, ideally within six hours, and this milk will then be given to your baby via a tube. The more you pump, the more your supply will establish. If you are unable to get enough milk for your baby, your NICU may have a milk bank of pasteurised, screened donor milk, or you may be able to source a

If you think your labour is starting prematurely. . .

Don't delay – contact your care provider immediately. Early labour is before 37 weeks. Signs can include: trickle of waters, increased vaginal discharge, cramps similar to period pains, vaginal bleeding, frequent need to urinate, nausea, vomiting, diarrhoea. If you feel worried or unwell in any way seek urgent medical attention. They can check you to establish that all is well with your baby. If you are in labour and are more than 35 weeks pregnant, they may let the birth go ahead, and if you are less than 35 weeks pregnant, they may try to stop the contractions or give steroid injections to help your baby breathe when they are born.

donor yourself via groups like Human Milk for Human Babies UK. Some, but not all, mums of premature babies report pressure to 'top up' with formula, so it might be wise to seek support and advice from your nearest lactation consultant (IBCLC), or one of the main breastfeeding organisations. For these and more links for parents of premature babies, see Resources.

What if... it's twins?

Finding out you are expecting twins comes as a huge shock to most pregnant couples! While some people may conceive twins through IVF, or have twins in the family, increasing their chances of having twins themselves, others find they are carrying two babies at once, totally out of the blue. Holy guacamole.

If this is you, try to stay calm. This may be hard without the option of a stiff drink, but – try. Twin births are normal and possible, and they happen to women, and women handle them!

'My experience was that everyone from my mum to the lady in Marks & Spencers was so highly anxious and negative about twins from the outset. "Double trouble, glad it's not me, oh how will you cope, my friend had twins and it was awful". Added to this, many of us find carrying two babies really hard work – by 37 weeks you can't move. Literally. So you're having to contend with all of that as well as normal pregnancy anxiety. I had my hospital bag packed and buggy delivered by 30 weeks in fear that something awful would happen. It was such a shock to get to 38 weeks and everything be fine, that I hadn't really had the foresight to think about the birth. Having twins is one of the best things that can ever happen to a person. Twins are amazing. I feel blessed every single day. It doesn't mean it's not challenging at times. It's the best though in so many ways. Double the cuddles, the love, the laughs, the friendship and that extra special connection.' Tricia Murray, mum of twins, Edinburgh

Being pregnant with twins will probably mean that you are offered more monitoring in your pregnancy than if you were expecting just the one baby. There are three kinds of twins: those that have their own placenta and membrane sac (known as di or DCDA), those that share a placenta but have their own sacs (mono or MCDA), and those that share a placenta and membrane sac (mono or MCMA).

All non-identical twins are DCDA, and one-third of identical twins are DCDA. The other two-thirds of identical twins are MCDA, and just 1 per cent of identical twins are MCMA.

Still with me? Right. Mums carrying MCDA and MCMA twins will be offered frequent scans and possibly care from a specialist, as there are higher risks of complications, whereas DCDA twins are the most straightforward kind and mums will therefore be offered scans every four weeks.

Obviously, having twins, and the kind of twins you are expecting, will also have an impact on the kind of birth you are offered. For any kind of twin birth, it will not be recommended that you have a home or birth centre birth, or a water birth, and you will also be advised to be induced at around 37 weeks for DCDA twins, and earlier for MCDA and MCMA twins.

In some hospitals, the 'twin package' extends beyond induction to include routine epidural and continuous electronic monitoring. Some women who are expecting twins (of either variety) decline induction and choose to have their babies at home, but it's unlikely this will happen within the NHS and you will need to speak to an Independent Midwife who has direct experience of twin birth. Others decide to decline induction but birth in hospital, but even this goes against NICE guidelines, which states that while there is no increased risk of adverse outcomes from induction of twins, continuing the pregnancy beyond 38 weeks increases the risk of stillbirth.

However, it's more likely than not that your labour will start spontaneously before this time – about 60 per cent of women pregnant with twins will start labour by 37 weeks. It's also interesting to try to find out what NICE means by 'increased risk of stillbirth' – increased from what to what? The World Health Organisation states that there is, 'insufficient evidence to issue a recommendation on induction of labour in women with an uncomplicated twin pregnancy at or near term'. And the wonderful Cochrane reviews of the evidence found that there was no advantage to induction at 37 weeks over expectant management (waiting and being monitored) in uncomplicated twin pregnancies. A separate Cochrane review also found no advantage to elective caesarean for uncomplicated twin pregnancies.

It seems that getting an accurate picture of the risk and making a truly informed choice is difficult with twins, and as usual you may also find that you get different advice or options depending on where in the world or even where in the country you live. And as usual, if you want to deviate from the standard path, for example by delaying or declining induction, or choosing out of hospital birth, then you will probably have to discuss this in depth with your caregivers and you may need to look for support from other women who have 'been there, done that' (social media is a great place to find them), or, if you are being told you are not allowed to make certain choices, try AIMS or Birthrights.

Felicity Jeffreys gave birth to twins in hospital in Cambridge

From my experience of being pregnant with twins I would say options are limited unless you have the confidence to ask and are sure of what birth you want. When I decided to refuse induction the consultants were pretty awful to me, telling me the babies would die and I was risking their lives. The first meeting I had was terrible, and it was hard for me to not feel like we were on different sides and fighting against each other. Then the supervisor of midwives (SOM) got involved and said she would help me to have the birth I wanted, and we revised my birth plan together.

It wasn't a surprise when I woke at 4am on 1 October with what I believed to be waters trickling out, because I had strongly visualised that this would happen, even to the time on the clock. I wanted to go into labour before a consultant meeting I had that very day, so I used every natural method I knew to make it happen and it did. I never question the mind-body connection and the power of thought. I was so excited to go into labour and felt like shouting, in fact I probably did shout, 'Bring it on'! I let Martin go back to sleep and came downstairs to phone my sister Letty, who was my other birth partner, and she said she would be over shortly. I remained pretty active for the next couple of hours using the ball and sofa for different positions, but was keen to know if the hospital had a room free with a pool. I knew they would allow me in at any time as it was twins! Luckily the room was free so I decided, as the surges were starting to feel a little stronger, we would leave.

We left the house around 7am, and I had surges fairly close together in the car. I sat in the back, I was breathing through them and in control. We parked and I had a few surges on the way from the car park, but I was enjoying them, knowing that this was all bringing me closer to my babies.

When we arrived I was so chuffed to see all the midwives gathered for a change of shift and each one of them was clutching my birth planning notes that had been emailed to them prior to me going into labour. This gave me a great feeling as these notes had been worked on for several weeks in partnership with the SOM and consultants. We got into the room with the pool, stuck my affirmations up and some pictures and they started filling the pool up. The midwife came to me and said she was in training and was this OK, but I had already decided that I didn't want a trainee present only for the simple fact that I didn't want talking in the room. I'm really nosy and would probably be trying to listen to what they were saying, which would be distracting for me. I ended up with another midwife, a male midwife who was absolutely fantastic; he had read my birth plan, always whispered to me and I felt like he was another support.

I got into the pool and was loving listening to my MP3s in my headphones, and the surges were getting more intense now. Martin and Letty would now and again engage with me, asking if I needed a drink, food or the toilet, and occasionally we would chat and have a laugh. I had radio monitoring as this was an agreement from my previous meetings, but the midwife was not happy that the readings were accurate so we took them off and he let me be in the pool for quite a while with no monitoring. Sometimes he would use a Doppler but I continued to be in my zone.

He then asked me to get out, so I did, another 30 minutes later! By now the surges were becoming much more intense and I requested mats and a ball. I put the ball on the bed and leant over it. I was hooked up to monitoring now but the leads were very long and gave me room to move and change position. I really felt that the first baby was bearing down and I was starting to get a pushing sensation with barely time to speak between surges. My midwife went to get a sandwich so another midwife took over, but I was sure he would miss it and told him so! I did get the feeling they thought I was nowhere near ready to birth. I knew I was though, so I continued to follow my body's lead.

I was standing up and occasionally leaning over the bed, and I was making a lot of animalistic noises, which felt natural. I think looking back I was going through transition – in that moment I had had enough – but I really felt that the baby was coming on the next surge and I did a poo. In that split second I wanted to cry because I thought the baby was coming and the midwife was now over the other side of the room! I had a big surge and Etta pretty much flew out, as I shouted, 'I'm having my baby!'. I caught her and felt I was going to drop her, so Letty grabbed her. The cord was really short so I then held her down by my tummy. I was euphoric, crying and laughing at the same time as I shuffled around looking at everyone's faces!

I knew I had a bit of time before the second baby. The midwives, now three in the room and my original midwife back, were rather speechless! They were keen to monitor baby two as they were worried he wouldn't find his way out, but I was so confident that he would and that it would be 20 minutes after his sister. I told them not to bother scanning me and I told them he was coming as the surges started again. By now I was on the bed as they instructed me for the scan; I couldn't move or change positions once the birth process started, but also I didn't want to move. I knew this wasn't the best position but everything felt as though it was happening and I still felt confident he would be here soon. It really wasn't many surges and he was here too, with a longer cord so he was able to come right up to my chest.

It was amazing I birthed two babies with no intervention or pain relief and having had a traumatic experience with my first born I can honestly say without my knowledge and preparation it would not have been like this at all. I spent the next hour and a half birthing the placentas, which had fused inside me, and bonding and breastfeeding with my babies, still in a bubble. I was already a mother but I felt different again, just like a shift in the universe. I had done something so natural and raw and it changed me, with so much love for my babies and feeling I had given them the best possible start.

What if... I have a low-lying placenta?

Some women are told at their 20-week scan that their placenta is 'low-lying'. This means that your placenta is lower down than normal, and, if it doesn't move in time for the birth, this can cause a problem. A low-lying placenta can overlap your cervix and, as you dilate, cause serious problems during labour such as bleeding.

The good news is that the majority of placentas that are low-lying at the 20-week scan will move out of the way in time for the birth. Research suggests that only about 1 in 600 placentas will refuse to budge (those dirty, rotten, low-lying scoundrels). If your placenta is low at your 20-week scan, you will be offered an extra scan to see how things have developed at about 32 weeks.

If your placenta is low in late pregnancy this is called 'placenta praevia'. You will be at a higher risk of complications, such as bleeding and reduced growth of your baby, so you will be offered extra monitoring. You will be told to rest and avoid sex and orgasms, and may have to spend the last weeks of pregnancy in hospital, because if you start bleeding or go into labour early, a caesarean may be immediately necessary. If you have already had a baby via caesarean, you may be at higher risk of a further complication known as 'placenta accreta'. This is when the placenta grows into the uterine wall and will not separate normally after the birth. This is a serious condition which can result in hysterectomy, but, like placenta praevia, it is thankfully rare. There are links to more information in Resources.

What if... I have pre-eclampsia?

Pre-eclampsia is a condition that affects blood flow to and from the placenta, and happens in about 5 per cent of pregnancies, although severe cases only develop in about 1–2 per cent of pregnancies. Pre-eclampsia usually develops after the 20th week of pregnancy (and very rarely, before), and the early signs are high blood pressure, or protein in your urine, which should be detected by your midwife at routine appointments. However, there are other symptoms, which as a pregnant woman, it's a very good idea to be aware of. These include:

- Heartburn or indigestion with pain after eating
- Swelling, for example of the feet
- Sudden weight gain

- Shoulder pain or pain when breathing deeply
- Malaise, or a feeling that something 'isn't right'
- Pain under the right side of the ribs
- Headache and changes in vision ('flashing lights')

Many of these may seem like common parts of pregnancy but it's important not to ignore them and to get checked immediately if you have any concerns.

The only 'cure' for pre-eclampsia is to give birth to your baby! If you are diagnosed with pre-eclampsia you will be carefully monitored and usually induced or offered a caesarean at around 37 or 38 weeks. Pre-eclampsia is a condition to take seriously, as it can lead to complications that can be life-threatening for you or your baby, such as eclampsia, and HELLP syndrome. For more info, see Resources.

What if... my labour is 'too long'?

Very long labours can be hard work. What seemed exciting when it first started can start to wear as thin as a fully-effaced cervix after 24 hours. Added to this, some long labours can be caused by awkwardly positioned babies (see page 133), which can make them more painful. Not fun.

It's unusual for a labour to be both long and relentless. If labour really is 'cracking on', then this normally means that you are dilating as you should and 'progressing' towards the pushing stage just fine.

Long labours tend to be very 'stop-start', especially to begin with. Most people who talk about 'being in labour for three days' are including this early phase in their calculations, rather than just talking about 'active labour' (the 'ramping up' and 'cracking on' stages, see pages 28-32), which tends to be an average of eight hours for first timers.

Houston, do we have a problem?

If your labour is long, you need to ask yourself one important question – is this a problem? If checks show that all is well with the baby, and if you are feeling strong and happy to keep going, then it could just be that this is the labour you were meant to have – and maybe you even want to take your time over it, let it build slowly, and relish the moment.

On the other hand, if you feel you are not coping, or you or others have concerns over your wellbeing or that of your baby, then maybe action needs to be taken. However, 'action', does not always mean an intravenous drip. There are tips elsewhere in this book for ways to get labour moving naturally, or cope when it doesn't.

 If your early labour feels a bit like a one-winged chicken trying to fly, see the tips on the 'long latent phase' on page 29. If you achieve take-off but are unable to stop circling the airport see Top Tips for Progress Failures on page 90.

What if... my labour is 'too short'?

What with all the horror stories of 'being in labour for four days', it might come as something of a shock to you if you're tidying the kitchen one minute and popping out a baby on the bathroom floor the next. This kind of very fast labour is known as 'precipitous', and is defined as such if you go from Zero to Hero in three hours or less. Precipitous labour is rare – it only happens in about 3 per cent of births – and it's both more likely, and easier to predict, for second or subsequent babies. If your first baby came quickly, it's likely (but not guaranteed) that your others will too.

Getting it all over with quickly might sound like a dream come true to some of us, and, if a short labour happens to you, you're likely to be told how 'lucky' you are by the other mums at the baby group. However, not everyone who has a fast labour feels this way – some women find the experience shocking or even traumatic.

There's nothing you can do to control the length of your labour; like many aspects of labour and birth it's one of those things that just seems to be written in the stars. However, just knowing that this could happen to you can help you to be more prepared for it. For example:

- Even if you are planning a birth centre or hospital birth, you might like to keep a little 'home birth kit' on hand, for example some old towels, a water bottle, camera and so on, just in case.
- If you have other children, make sure you have made arrangements with someone who can take care of them quickly and easily.
- Talk with your partner or birth partner about what you might do if labour is fast. How far do you live from the hospital? Will you still go in the car, or stay home and call a midwife or ambulance?
- Get your partner to prepare themselves for a quick labour too. Nudge them into doing a little homework, so they know what to expect, and make sure they know what your wishes are.

- Be aware that paramedics are not midwives and may not be as up to speed on current best practice, for example delayed cord clamping or skin-to-skin. Make sure you or your partner speak up if you think they are cutting the cord too soon or doing anything else you would rather they did not do.
- Remember your rights: if you have a fast, unplanned home birth (sometimes called a BBA – born before arrival of the midwife), then you don't have to automatically transfer to hospital, although you will probably want to do so should there be any concerns about you or your baby's wellbeing.

What if... the cord is around my baby's neck?

This often tops the list of people's fears about childbirth, but in fact, it really needn't. For starters, it's extremely common – 'nuchal cord', as it is known, occurs in around one third of all births. Many people have the impression that a baby can become 'strangled' by its cord being around its neck, but of course this simply isn't possible, since a baby does not take their first breath until after they are born, and all the oxygen they need is supplied via the cord itself. During the birth, the uterus is contracting and baby, uterus and placenta are all making 'downwards motions' together, so the image that some people have of the cord working like a 'noose' as the baby moves down just isn't accurate. Having a nuchal cord is also not a reason for early clamping or cord cutting. If your baby is born with the cord around their neck, you, your midwife or your birth partner can gently unloop it and it is unlikely to cause any problem whatsoever.

What if... I want to opt out of certain procedures or make choices that my midwives and doctors do not recommend?

You have the right to accept or decline everything that is offered to you in your maternity care. Under law, pregnant women are afforded the same rights as anyone else to refuse any aspect of medical care, even if this poses a risk to themselves or their baby. Just as you can't be forced to have surgery to remove a kidney – even if this might save your life or the life of your unwell twin – you cannot be forced to undergo any procedure when you are pregnant or in labour.

Of course, you – like the vast majority of women – will want to make the best and safest choices for yourself and your baby. However, the best and safest choice will not always be the same choice for each woman, and if you wish to make an informed decision to decline any aspect of your treatment, you have the right to do so.

You must be asked for your consent for anything that happens to you in birth and you must not feel that you are being given one-sided information about this choice or that your care provider is strongly biased towards your making one choice over another. Nor must you feel like you are being coerced or even bullied into a particular choice. Consent given in these circumstances is not legally valid and your healthcare provider may be liable to be prosecuted for such serious offences as trespass against the person, or battery.

If there is an emergency and you are unable to make your wishes known, for example if you are unconscious, then treatment may be given without your consent. However, if there is a next of kin available, they should be consulted and involved in decisions.

You also have the right to choose where you give birth to your baby, so long as you have mental capacity to make your own decisions. Even if you are told you are 'high risk', you can still decide to birth at home, and your care providers should work with you to put this plan into place. MLUs can be difficult for higher-risk women to access – but anecdotally such women often find the birth centre door mysteriously opens if they start to talk about home birth.

Once your baby has been born, the person with 'parental responsibility' (this is usually the mother) is also entitled to decline any aspect of care on their behalf.

Can this be challenged?
In spite of the fact that the profile of human rights in childbirth continues to be raised, there are still many situations where women find that, although they are clear about their choices, these choices are deemed unacceptable by birth professionals.

Language that suggests that the balance of power is tipped in favour of the hospital may be used, for example:

'You are not allowed to have a home birth if your last birth was a caesarean.'

'We can't admit you unless we know your dilation so unfortunately we do need to examine you.'

'All premature babies receive this injection.'

This sort of language is wrongly weighted and misleading; however, in day-to-day reality it happens and it can be very difficult to challenge. Know that, whatever maternity choices you wish to make, the law is on your side and supports your right to make those choices, even if they are not compliant with hospital policy and even if they are not the choice recommended by your care providers.

The circumstances under which your choices can validly be challenged are rare. If you lack mental capacity, or if there is a child protection concern, the professionals involved in your care can raise questions about your decision-making, but this will still be subject to rigorous process and assessment and it cannot be decided by any one individual that you lack capacity or that you are placing your child at risk.

More information can be found on the Birthrights website (see Resources).

What if... I'm told 'you're not allowed'?

Beverley Beech is Chair of the Association for Improvement in Maternity Services (AIMS), who frequently support women in this situation.

'Am I allowed?' is a common question that women ask, as many think that they are required to do whatever the staff advise. However, the NHS and health professionals are there to provide a service – not to dictate what women must or must not do. They have a professional duty to support your decisions. If you are told that you 'have to' do something, or that you 'are not allowed', you could consider saying that you are aware of your right to make your own decisions about your body and your baby, and your right to decline treatment and advice if you wish.

To access support if you are told 'You're not allowed' contact the AIMS helpline or Birthrights (see Resources).

What if... my baby is big?

Growing a giant baby that's too big to get out: could this be every pregnant woman's deepest fear? Certainly it seems like we're all slightly obsessed with the topic, as not a week goes by without an 'eye-watering' birth story making the rounds in the media.

As every woman who's ever had a baby will know, one of the first questions everyone asks you after the birth is, 'How much did they weigh?' If your answer is less than seven pounds they will reply, 'Oh, not too bad then!'; anything over that number and everyone says, 'Blimey', and pulls the sort of face they usually only reserve for groin injury stories after the game on Saturday.

If you're told that you're having a big baby, you might want to factor that into your plans – or you may not. Giving birth to a big baby vaginally is possible, and worrying excessively about your baby's size can potentially cause more trouble than the size in itself. Once it's suspected that your baby may be larger than average, you are more likely to be anxious about giving birth, and your care providers are more likely to offer you monitoring and interventions in labour, which in turn can increase your risk of caesarean and other complications.

Unfortunately, and regardless of what you may be told, scans are not an accurate way to predict your baby's size, so the idea of a 'late reassurance scan' is pretty misleading. Many studies have looked at the accuracy of both scans and physical exams to predict baby size, and the verdict is that these methods have such big margins for error that they are unlikely to be of much use. If your care provider is telling you that they know for sure you are expecting a larger than average baby, you may like to ask them for the evidence for this.

Almost two thirds of very big babies (4.5kg or more) are born vaginally. Larger babies have an increased risk of shoulder dystocia (when the head is born, but the shoulders are stuck), which can – in around 1 in 1,000 births – cause something called brachial plexus palsy, nerve damage that can be temporary or, even more rarely (in about 15 per cent of that 1 in 1,000 figure), permanent.

Shoulder dystocia is impossible to predict, and it can and does happen to smaller babies too. The majority of cases of shoulder dystocia can be resolved by skilled care providers, whether you are at home or in hospital, most often by manoeuvres like McRoberts (where you lie on your back and your legs are pushed outwards and up towards your chest), or the Gaskin manoeuvre (where you are helped on to all-fours).

My own big babies

Women like me get the best reaction when revealing their baby's weight – it can only be described as a stunned silence, followed by just one word: 'Whoah'. I'm a narrow-hipped girl who can just about squeeze into size 8 jeans, so I was as shocked as the next person when my second baby tipped the scales at 10lb 4oz.

Perhaps more shocking still, the birth was easy! That is, if the word easy can ever be applied to birth – it certainly did smart a bit. So when I say 'easy', what I mean is, it happened at home, it didn't hurt so much that I felt I needed pain relief (not even gas and air), the 'pushing' bit lasted about five minutes, and I didn't need any stitches.

There was no anxiety in my pregnancy about the size of my baby. I had a big bump, but according to the midwife's tape measure it was bang on target. So we breezed into a home water birth feeling confident, not knowing what a total chubster was silently biding her time in my ever-expanding uterus.

The anxiety – entirely absent for her delivery – came afterwards. My GP was the first to raise it: in his surgery her birth weight came up in conversation and he told me that were I ever to have another, 'they would not let me have another home birth'.

Having given birth twice I felt confident enough to question this. Pregnant for the third (and final) time in 2013, I sought a variety of views on the safety of another home delivery, including a senior consultant's, and the unanimous verdict seemed to be: if you did it once you can do it again. So I did – my 9lb 11oz boy was born at home, and it was 'easy'; although if you'd used that word near me any time in the final hour of the labour you'd still be walking with a limp.

The positions you adopt during labour can reduce your risk of shoulder dystocia – which is tellingly sometimes called 'bed dystocia' by midwives. Remember – being flat on your back on the bed decreases the size of your pelvis by 30 per cent – and this is not going to help you give birth with ease regardless of your baby's size. If you read the birth stories of women who have birthed big babies without trouble, it's interesting to note how many of them report giving birth upright, kneeling, on all-fours or in a birth pool. They are rarely, if ever, on their back.

Louisa Aldridge's third baby Connie was 9lb 1oz. 'All my babies have been about the same size, and quite big and I am quite a small person: 5ft 4in and a dress size 8. I've been active in all my labours and I gave birth to Connie at home in a pool.'

Louisa did worry about big babies, especially during her first pregnancy when people would remark on the size of her bump: 'Like many others, I assumed it was impossible to push a big baby out without doing yourself some kind of damage. But I read childbirth guru Ina May Gaskin's advice – it's all about increasing blood flow to the pelvic area, making the tissues super stretchy – and it worked!'

Louisa also paid attention to her birth environment, with 'dim lighting, a loving vibe and a warm pool', something that doula and founder of Tell Me A Good Birth Story Natalie Meddings says is vital:

'Babies do seem to be getting bigger, which is not a problem in itself as women don't tend to grow a baby they are unable to get out. The real problem is that this is happening in tandem with a system that very often ignores women's physiological needs and they are still being urged onto the bed. They may be denied the deep darkness and profound privacy needed to enable total disinhibition and complete release of every tiny muscle in that area to facilitate the passage of a baby of any size, not just the big ones! If we carry on ignoring what women really need, then bigger babies are going to cause problems.'

If you are worried about birthing a big baby, then the best thing you can do is have the kind of active labour and oxytocin-enhancing birth environment that works better for everyone. Remember that many women who have had different sized babies report that the bigger ones were 'easier' – perhaps because of their stronger gravitational pull!

What if... I am rhesus negative?

Many of us aren't even aware of our blood group, but when you're pregnant, you will probably agree to have your blood tested, and you will be alerted if your blood group is 'rhesus negative'. Only about 15 per cent of us have rhesus-negative blood, which means that blood cells have a substance known as 'D antigen' on their surface. Nothing abnormal, and nothing to worry about.

However, if your partner is not rhesus negative too, this can mean that your baby, like him, will be rhesus positive. Again, this is not in itself a problem, unless something happens in your pregnancy or birth that causes your blood and your baby's blood to mix. This event is sometimes called 'sensitisation' and if it happens, the body creates a template for the production of antibodies that it can use again in future pregnancies.

Even a tiny amount of your baby's rhesus positive blood mixing with your rhesus negative blood can cause this sensitisation. It's highly unlikely to happen, but the likelihood increases with any event that might cause bleeding, for example, tests such as chorionic villus sampling, amniocentesis, or a trauma such as a car accident. Interventions during labour carry a much-reduced risk, but might include forceps delivery, caesarean, or accidental tearing of the cord. Be aware that sensitisation can happen during termination, miscarriage, or ectopic pregnancy too, so if you are rhesus negative and have experienced any of these events, discuss this with your healthcare provider.

Once sensitised, your body may produce antibodies against the rhesus positive cells, known as 'Anti-D antibodies'. This is very unlikely to affect your current pregnancy, but if you have subsequent children they too may be rhesus positive. Your body may trigger an immune response, sometimes called 'rhesus incompatibility'. Anti-D antibodies can cross the placenta and destroy the baby's blood cells, which can cause miscarriage or stillbirth, or a condition at birth known as rhesus disease, or haemolytic disease of the newborn (not to be confused with haemorrhagic disease of the newborn, which is associated with vitamin K deficiency, see page 114). This can cause anaemia and jaundice, and in rare cases, can be fatal.

The NICE guidelines therefore recommend that all rhesus negative pregnant women have an injection known as 'Anti-D' at 28 weeks. If any traumatic event occurs that could cause sensitisation, another shot of Anti-D is given. At birth, cord blood is tested to establish your baby's blood group, and if they are found to be rhesus positive, you are offered a final injection of Anti-D within 72 hours of the birth. (Note: you can have optimal cord clamping if you are rhesus negative, see page 107.)

Trials are currently taking place in the UK of a new system that tests the baby's blood group in utero, thus eliminating the need for rhesus-negative women carrying a rhesus-negative baby to have the shot. Until this test is widely available, Anti-D will continue to be given 'prophylactically' – which is the medical word meaning 'preventatively' or 'just in case'. In other words, you might not need Anti-D, but you get it anyway.

Some women are happy to consent to all injections of Anti-D, while others take some but not all, or decline completely. Anti-D is made from a blood product, so if you have religious beliefs that conflict with receiving products of this nature, or you are concerned about possible risks, you may wish to decline. At the moment there are no known risks of accepting the injection but, while Anti-D is known to cross the placenta, there have been no studies of the long-term effects of the product on the baby.

For this reason some women decline Anti-D in pregnancy, but accept it after the birth if their baby is found to be rhesus positive. Still others only accept the shot if there is a traumatising event in their pregnancy that may cause sensitisation. Women who know for certain that they absolutely don't want to have another baby in the future sometimes decline the postnatal dose, as the only purpose of this is to protect subsequent pregnancies. As always, the task is one of balancing risk and making the choice that feels right for you.

What if... my baby is breech?

If your baby is 'breech', it means that instead of being 'head down', they have their head in your ribs and their bottom or feet near the exit. You're probably feeling worried, but I urge you not to adopt the 'rabbit in the headlights' approach – there are loads of really proactive things you can do.

First of all, how pregnant are you?

If you are less than 34 weeks and have been told your baby is breech, there is every possibility that they will flip into the more favoured head-down position: only about 3 to 4 per cent of babies are still in the breech position at term.

There are also active methods that all women – not just those who are worried about breech – can undertake to encourage their baby to find a favourable position: see optimal foetal positioning, page 133).

Past 34 weeks?

There is still a lot you can do.

- Try some of the techniques suggested by Spinning Babies to 'flip a breech' (see Resources). These involve getting yourself in various physical positions to use gravity and your own body to encourage baby to move.
- Place warmth (like a hot water bottle) where you want baby to move towards. You can also try playing music or using dad's voice to encourage baby to move in a certain direction. Or if you're feeling a little more ruthless, place a cold object (like a bag of frozen peas), where you want them to move away from!
- Try moxibustion: this is an acupuncture technique that sounds utterly bizarre but is claimed to have good results. A small stick of incense is lit and held over an acupuncture point. It's non-invasive and doesn't hurt. Worth a try.
- Other alternative therapies such as osteopathy, homeopathy, herbs and massage are also worth considering, although you must find a practitioner who is skilled in pregnancy and preferably understands breech.

Past 36 weeks and still breech?

You may be offered an ECV. This procedure – External Cephalic Version – is done by an obstetrician in the hospital, usually between 37 weeks and term, and involves being given a drug to relax your muscles, and then the doctor trying to gently move the baby into the head-down position. ECV has around a 50 per cent success rate, but this does vary widely between practitioners, so it is worth asking what outcomes your specific hospital or doctor has and 'shopping around' to find the person with the best success rates. ECV carries a very small risk (about 1 in 200) of causing complications, such as placental bleeding or changes in the baby's heartbeat, which will result in you needing an immediate caesarean.

If your baby 'flips'...

If your ECV or any other technique you try is successful in persuading your baby to turn head down, then please don't sink back on the sofa in relief! You need to keep active – brisk walking daily is good – to get baby's head to settle into your pelvis. As long as baby stays head down, there is now no reason why you should not have a straightforward vaginal birth in the setting of your choice. You should be able to tell what position your baby is in from the location of the kicks, but if you are not sure, your midwife or doctor can check for you.

If nothing works and you have a breech baby for sure...

At this point the options can seem fairly Rock vs Hard Place, and I first of all want to give you a hug. OK. Better? Nope... so, as always, information is power.

First of all, a little background. It's likely that you are being offered a caesarean for your breech baby, and you might be wondering – what did women do before this option was so readily available, or even before scans came along to tell us for sure the position of our baby? The answer is, they had their babies vaginally, and their midwives usually knew how to deal with the situation.

Breech birth requires highly specialised midwifery skills, but in recent years, in particular due to a piece of research published in 2000 known as the Hannah or Term Breech Trial, caesarean birth has become the default option. The Hannah trial has since been called into question, but in the meantime many midwives have had little or no experience of vaginal breech birth – and the specialist skills required have been lost.

World renowned experts like Mary Cronk and Jane Evans – midwives who specialise in vaginal breech birth – describe it as 'another variation of normal', and use the phrase 'hands off the breech'. A successful breech birth, they argue, is one where the birth assistants are 'hands off', allowing mother to follow her own instincts, which will almost always call her to position herself on her hands and knees. Such midwives will only ever touch the labouring woman or the emerging baby if it is absolutely necessary, and in these cases they have the specialist understanding to safely assist the baby out.

However, the hands-off approach is not always understood in UK hospitals, where you may find you are being offered a very 'managed' birth in theatre, with continuous monitoring, epidural, lithotomy (on your back, feet in stirrups), episiotomy and probably forceps.

So – I suggest two courses of action. Either choose vaginal breech birth and go Birthzilla in your hunt for information. Find out what your local doctors offer, discuss with them the fine details of their experience and their approach. Explore what other hospitals or units in your area might offer. Talk to other women in local birth groups and use the great pool of knowledge available on social media in groups like Breech Birth UK. Hunt down local birth professionals like doulas and antenatal teachers to pick their brains, and consider the option of an independent midwife who may be more likely to have the skills you need.

Alternatively, choose caesarean and shock the pants off your local hospital with your long list of exquisite demands. Make it the best, gentlest, most woman-centred experience you can, and do what you need to do to make your peace with that.

What if... there is something 'wrong' with my baby?

Not all babies are well during pregnancy or after birth – yet another reason to dislike the phrase 'a healthy baby is all that matters'. For some parents or parents-to-be, there will be difficult times if their baby is discovered to be poorly in some way. This may happen during routine antenatal appointments, such as scans, or, less commonly, you may discover at birth that your baby has a physical problem or disability. Your baby may also be unwell and need special care, for example if they are born prematurely, if they have jaundice, if they are have a low birth weight, or if they have an infection. All of these situations can be extremely difficult for parents and parents-to-be, but there is a lot of support and information available that may make this time easier for you. See Resources for links for specific situations.

What if... I lose my baby?

Writing this book, I faced a dilemma. Do I talk about loss? Of course, I absolutely don't want to make you feel worried at a time that may already be filled with anxiety. But on the other hand, I don't want to sweep the issue of loss under the carpet. Because it happens. I desperately hope it doesn't happen to you. But it happens. And it's been swept under the carpet for decades, often to the great detriment of those who experience it.

There is no line in the sand that dictates when a developing baby starts to matter to a woman. Usually, the process of bonding with a child begins before they are born, but everyone is different. Regardless of how you feel or think you feel about the life developing inside you, you will probably still find losing your baby at any stage of your pregnancy a very tough experience.

In our culture, miscarriage and stillbirth have long been taboo topics, and women have been encouraged not to 'indulge' too much in the resulting emotional fall-out. We are now learning that insisting that everyone keeps quiet in the wake of baby loss does not mean

Birth matters

It's often assumed that, if parents discover that their baby has a problem that means they are incompatible with life, that they don't care about how that baby is born. While for some people this may be true, I have also had the privilege of speaking to several parents who have lost babies, for whom the birth experience itself was a source of great tenderness and comfort in the difficult days, weeks and years that followed.

One such mother was Natalie, from Kent, who discovered that her baby had Potter's Syndrome, a rare disease meaning he had no kidneys and would therefore die at birth or shortly after. Having planned a home birth, Natalie initially thought she would abandon this idea and have the recommended hospital termination, followed by an induced birth under epidural. However, after taking a few weeks to consider the decision, she decided to continue with her plans for a home birth.

'If my baby had any chance of survival then I would not want to be at home, nor if I needed medical help', she told me. 'But for sadness alone, I felt there was not much the hospital could offer.' Natalie describes the last remaining weeks of her pregnancy as a very special time in which she connected to her baby and even read him children's books aloud. She carried him to 43 weeks – highly unusual in a baby with his condition – and had the home birth she had hoped for throughout her pregnancy. 'The birth was wonderful and I never felt scared, overcome with any negative feeling, nor even cried throughout the birth and meeting my baby. It was the best and most monumental part of a sad story'.

To other parents in similar situations, Natalie says, 'My advice is to take as much time as you need to make a decision about your choices. Express your love and grief to the fullest, and you will move forward with no regrets. All parenthood of any child involves letting go, and this is the ultimate letting go, doing as much for your child as you can, but then knowing you can do no more. All has been achieved, all that the child needed. We looked after him till he "left home".'

that the feelings simply 'go away', and that – quite the opposite – being allowed time and space to grieve can be tremendously helpful and mean that people feel they can find 'closure' and move on with their lives.

If you lose a baby at any stage of pregnancy, you have a right to mourn this loss. It can be very helpful to do as much as possible to remember your baby and honour their existence, however brief. If you lose your baby after 24 weeks this is defined as 'stillbirth', and hospitals are now much better at helping parents 'make memories'. Some offer 'cuddle cots' so that you can take as long as you need to say goodbye. Often you will be helped to bathe your baby, dress them, make hand and footprints, and take photographs. This will be a very painful and sad time, but parents also report this time spent with their baby to be hugely comforting as they move forwards with their grief.

Losing a baby before 24 weeks is termed miscarriage and can sometimes – insensitively – be treated as a 'lesser' loss than stillbirth. As with all difficult life events, you will find ways to cope that are right for you. Although there are no UK national standards for what should happen after miscarriage, you do still have a right to take your baby home, or to have a funeral service, a cemetery burial, or to have the ashes after a cremation. You may have to ask for this and it may not be offered, although hopefully this is changing.

Regardless of what stage of pregnancy you experience loss, you may also find it helpful to do something meaningful like planting a tree or creating a special garden as a place to remember.

You can find more support for baby loss in the Resources.

What if... my baby has Down's Syndrome or another chromosomal condition?

Around the 10th to 14th week of pregnancy you will be offered a screening test for Down's Syndrome (Trisomy 21). This test is called the 'combined test' because it uses results from a blood test and combines them with information from your 12-week scan to give you an assessment of the likelihood of your baby having Down's Syndrome. The combined test also assesses your risk of two other chromosomal conditions, Edwards' Syndrome (Trisomy 18) and Patau's Syndrome (Trisomy 13).

If you are further into your pregnancy than 14 weeks, you will be offered other tests instead to assess the likelihood of Down's, Edwards' or Patau's. Both these tests and the combined test are non-invasive and none of them will give you a definitive answer. They will tell you if you are 'low risk' or 'high risk'. If the chance of your baby having Down's, Edwards' or Patau's is less than 1 in 150, this is considered a low-risk result and more than 95 per cent of screenings will fall into this category.

If your test result is higher than 1 in 150, this is considered a high risk and you will be offered 'diagnostic tests' that can give a definitive 'yes or no' answer, such as Chorionic Villus Sampling (CVS) and amniocentesis. These tests carry about a 1 per cent risk of causing miscarriage.

A new test, called NIPT (Non-Invasive Prenatal Test), sometimes known by brand names such as Harmony, is also available, although at the moment it is not the standard NHS offering and you will probably need to pay for the test privately. This test, which looks at DNA, is also 'screening' rather than 'diagnostic', and you will still be advised to have an amniocentesis if your test is positive. However, the NIPT is thought to be much more accurate in its prediction of chromosomal abnormalities than the existing tests, meaning you are less likely to have to consider the option of amniocentesis if it is not necessary.

All these screenings and tests are optional, and it's important to consider what a diagnosis would actually mean to you, your partner and your family, before you enter into the difficult territory of decision-making that comes with each opportunity for testing. Tests may be offered with the promise of 'peace of mind', but remember that this only tends to come with the result you want to hear.

If you do consent to screening and a diagnostic test confirms that your baby has Down's, Edwards' or Patau's, you still have choices. A confirmation of Edwards' or Patau's is, unfortunately, the most difficult result to receive. Babies with these conditions often do not survive pregnancy or live for very long after birth, although some do live for longer. It's important to stress that this result is very different to a diagnosis of Down's Syndrome. Parents of babies with Edwards' or Patau's often choose termination, but some prefer to continue with the pregnancy in the hopes of meeting their baby, even if only for a short time. Either way, this is a very difficult time, and you will need support and more information from professionals and charities such as SoftUK and Emily's Star.

If your baby is confirmed to have Down's Syndrome, the outlook

Hayley Goleniowska, whose daughter Natty has Down's Syndrome, offers her perspective

I think society has built up a fearful image of Down's Syndrome and I was certainly wrong before I knew Natty. Everything I thought I knew about the condition has been proved wrong. Everything.

With a diagnosis of Down's, termination is often assumed to be the only route. Unfortunately, many women report loaded language at their medical appointments, such as 'risk', 'I'm sorry', 'chromosomal abnormality', 'bad news', 'burden', and, although many professionals do give unbiased support, at worst some doctors and midwives are reported to give personal opinion: 'I wouldn't have this baby if I were you', 'I can't treat you if you continue', 'Your marriage will be over if you don't end this nonsense now', 'We need to act fast' and so on. Added to this, much of the info given out on Down's Syndrome is very old, based on shorter life expectancy from 50 years ago and doesn't take into account early intervention that means children can lead independent lives with support.

When a diagnosis of Down's Syndrome is given parents need time to think and process, consider their options, perhaps talk to a learning disability nurse, consult various charities or meet a family to understand the challenges and joys of parenting a child with Down's Syndrome. Booking someone in for a termination the next day as the assumed only route must change.

What's also important is that parents are given a human picture of the baby they are carrying too. It's all too often a medicalised view of Down's Syndrome, with simply a list of co-morbidities. It's easy to forget that each child is a completely unique individual with their own likes and dislikes, a full range of emotions – a person who will have more in common with their own family and community than with other children with Down's Syndrome.

I feel extraordinarily privileged to be Natty's mum. She has taught us to slow down and appreciate the details in life, to live in the moment with honesty and enthusiasm. She has taught us that we cannot plan for everything, and that perfection comes in many forms. I would not change one single thing about her, no, not even her extra chromosome. We truly are the lucky ones.

I will not judge you, whatever path you take, but I know that there is no test for the bright, feisty, gorgeous young lady in our family. The one who annoys the hell out of her big sister but is always the first to warmly hug a sad friend. The one who rides horses, swims like a fish and knows the lyrics to every Mary Poppins song. The one who is always centre of attention at parties or school events. The one who lives life to the full. The one who climbs into bed every morning, strokes my face and says 'Mummy, you are beautiful.' To which I reply, 'So are you. Beautiful. And perfect in every way.'

is usually very different. Each child with Down's Syndrome is different and has different needs, but a child with Down's Syndrome can usually be supported to live a fulfilling life, with levels of independence that are appropriate to them, and a life expectancy of around 60 or beyond. Speak to your healthcare providers about the specifics of your particular case, but as always, bear in mind that the choice is completely yours.

What if... I don't get the birth I want?

There is a lot of talk around disappointment when it comes to birth, especially in the media, who often like to blame any difficult postnatal feelings on the woman herself: if only she hadn't got her silly hopes up, she wouldn't be finding things so tough. This starts another rather destructive cycle in which women either don't plan for birth in the misguided belief that it's pointless, or do so but then spend the rest of eternity thinking that their postnatal sorrow could have been avoided if only they hadn't bought all those tea-lights.

The reality is much, much more complicated than this. First of all, all human beings are entitled to feel a bit miffed if they have a dream about something and it doesn't turn out that way. It's normal to feel let down, sad, or even a bit gutted if you don't get what you wanted.

Added to this, the birth experience is important to women. This is a big moment in our lives, where a brand new human being who we will love more than we ever thought possible, actually comes through us and out of us and into the world! This is big stuff! It's bigger than a holiday of a lifetime, it's arguably bigger than a wedding day – so of course we are entitled to have a vision of how we would like it to be and to feel a bit disenchanted if it's nothing like how we imagined.

But whereas when a wedding day goes wrong we might be looking at a bit of rain or an embarrassing trip-up on the dance floor, when birth doesn't go to plan this often means we've had an experience that may have been frightening or just downright traumatic. So as well as disappointment, many more difficult feelings can be added into the mix of postnatal emotions, and there may be physical scars that need time to heal as well.

It's important to distinguish between postnatal 'sorrow', and postnatal depression or PTSD. It is normal to feel a range of 'negative' feelings after you have had a baby, and this does not mean that there is anything wrong with you or that you love your baby any less. It is just 'real life', and I know you know this because you are a grown-up and a mother and you are handling it all in your own way. However, if these difficult feelings start to feel more than just a 'normal reaction to a tough time'; if you feel desperate, out of control, traumatised or unable to cope, I urge you to seek professional support. You can read more about postnatal emotions on pages 285 to 294.

You also have the right to make a formal complaint about the maternity care you received. If you think you want to do this, it is a good idea to write down as much as you can remember about your birth as soon as you can, and also to request a copy of your maternity notes. You may also want to report an individual practitioner to their professional body, or take legal action. For more information on this, visit the Birthrights website (see Resources).

If you don't think you need professional help, and you don't want to make a complaint, it is still a good idea to talk about your birth with someone you trust. For more on this, see the section on debriefing from birth on page 287.

Please honour your feelings of disappointment and the loss of the birth you had hoped for. In their attempts to console you, many people may tell you to focus on your baby, and while this is well-meant, it may make you feel like you are being selfish for caring about what your actual experience of birth was like. Motherhood is a time when we are supposed to be feeling fulfilled and skipping through cornfields with our baby on our hip, and we might feel like we are letting the side down if we're just not in the mood for that. It's also possible to find motherhood really enjoyable and fulfilling and feel upset about your birth experience (just as you can have a 'dream birth' and then struggle emotionally with the transition to motherhood).

Having and feeling a smorgasbord of complex, varying and even opposing emotions is a normal part of being human. Accept yourself in the emotional state you find yourself in right now, and know that this will change and evolve as all things do. Just as you are allowed to make the choices you wish to make in birth, you are also allowed to feel any way you wish to about it afterwards.

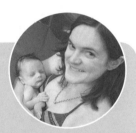

Rebirthing: Sarah tells of how 'rebirthing' in water helped her emotional healing following her son's difficult birth

March 2013: the month my world turned upside down. Three years earlier I'd had a fantastic home water birth with my daughter Lydia, and I naturally hoped for, and to some extent probably expected, the same second time around. I was healthy, well informed, had an incredibly positive approach to birth, and we had also had an independent midwife to support us. What could possibly go wrong?

Unfortunately the reality was rather different. We had a rocky pregnancy, with a diagnosis of talipes (club foot) and possible growth restriction. Then, at just past 39 weeks pregnant, I felt my baby's movements slow, and my instincts told me that something wasn't right.

I soon found myself in the hospital, making the only choice I could, to have an emergency caesarean. Jasper was born weighing a little over five and a half pounds, was very floppy and covered with thick meconium, inside and out. It scares me to think about it, but I know we got him out just in time.

An emergency caesarean was clearly the polar opposite of everything we hoped for in Jasper's birth. Instead of coming into the world in a warm birthing pool at home, he was plucked from me in a bright, unfamiliar operating theatre. Despite knowing I was making the right decision, it was the scariest night of my life – our little boy was so, so close to not surviving. Jasper spent eight days in NICU before we were finally able to come home where we belong.

My midwife Jo suggested that we might like to consider having a 'rebirth' for Jasper in the birthing pool once we had settled back at home. My initial reaction was sceptical – why would I want to upset myself with thoughts of the gentle birth that Jasper and I could no longer have?

I decided, though, to go into it with an open mind. Nine days after we came home from hospital, my husband Ben inflated and filled the pool just as he had planned to do when I went into labour. I climbed into the pool and instantly felt calm and happy. Jasper was passed to me, and seconds after touching the water, fell fast asleep. We spent time in the water together, listening to the special songs I had hoped to give birth to, and I whispered words of love and comfort to Jasper. I repeated a line that Ben and I had written into our wedding vows nearly seven years earlier – 'We will catch you if you fall and help you live your dreams'.

My initial worries about 'rebirthing' Jasper had left me, and although it was an emotional and at times sad experience, I know I will forever be glad that we got the birthing pool back out and spent that precious time giving Jasper a calm, wonderful rebirth. Jasper's birth and the surrounding events were incredibly difficult, and will always be a part of me. But alongside those memories I will now forever be able to think back to how he slept in my arms in the birthing pool, and how I looked down at my precious, miracle boy and started to believe for the first time that the emotional wounds from his birth and early days might one day heal.

❧ Chapter 13 ❧
Birth of a Mother

The baby is born, now what?!

If the time when we are waiting for birth is our Zwischen, then what should we call the time after? Those first few crazy hours, days, weeks, when we are not only getting to know our baby, but also, essentially, starting a whole new life, a whole new identity as 'mother' or 'father' or 'parent'? This change is on such an epic level that I'm going to go for Verwandlung, which basically translates as metamorphosis.

I like Verwandlung because, whether intentionally or not, it sounds a bit like, wandering, wondering, and wonder, and I felt there was a lot of all three of these things for me in my first few months of motherhood. I was exploring uncharted territory, full of questions, a bit lost, a bit worried and a bit amazed. There's also a really strong parallel here with the metamorphic journey from caterpillar to butterfly, which from the outside looks pretty poetic, but in reality involves the bug literally digesting itself into liquid and emerging finally (with what must be surely be a mixture of triumph, surprise and perhaps a small helping of smugness), from the resulting soup.

The interesting thing about caterpillars, though, is that the plans for butterfly status were always in place. Each one of them has something known as 'imaginal discs', parts of themselves that already know how to be eyes, wings, and legs, and even though the rest of the caterpillar becomes liquidised, the imaginal discs are still strong and still there, holding their knowing and slowly releasing the code for change.

I hope this chapter helps you as you enter your Verwandlung. It will give you some information from the outside, but it's perhaps important to remember that much of what you need to know is already within you. Your imaginal discs are in place, and eventually, in what may now seem like an impossible feat, you will emerge from the soup and take flight.

All about... Babymoons

It's a skill we've lost: just 'being there'. In our busy modern world, we often feel like we have to be 'doing', rather than 'being' – we have to have some kind of output to show for our time, we have to be productive.

Time spent with a newborn baby can feel like treading water. Where once by 11am we would have been dressed up smart and planning lunch with colleagues, with our newborns we find ourselves still in our sick-spattered pyjamas, eating crusts straight from the breadbin and washing them down with a cold cuppa.

This can feel like failure. Then, to make matters worse, we scroll through our newsfeed and see women being showered with praise for their amazing 'post-baby bodies' – there they are on the red carpet looking dazzling and just like they never had a baby. Their figure, their career, their social life: they got it all back, and fast.

It hasn't always been this way. In other cultures, and in different historical times, women have been worshipped for their ability to grow, birth and sustain a little life, and, in particular in the first few weeks after birth, encouraged to do absolutely nothing else but hold, feed and love their baby.

These traditions, now largely lost in the West, encourage us to feel that holding, nurturing and 'being there' for our newborns are activities of real value, not just to our baby but to our wider community and society. In many cultures, the babymoon lasts around 40 days, and during this time, the mother and newborn are fed special foods and cared for by others, and the mother is exempt from whatever her normal 'duties' may have been. In China, this time is called the 'golden month'.

Somehow the word 'babymoon', first used by Sheila Kitzinger, has recently been misappropriated to mean a fancy holiday taken during a couple's first pregnancy, a sort of 'final fling' before they start their new life as parents. If you really want to do this, and don't mind having to abstain from the all-inclusive cocktail menu, go for it. But I'd encourage you to try and have some time after the baby has been born too, when you take the pressure off to achieve anything other than wall-to-wall snuggles.

When you're making your birth plan, consider making a Babymoon Plan as well. There are many ways that you and your partner can plan for this time in advance and make it extra special, and your friends and family can support you too. Some couples even choose to have a short period of time – usually between 24 hours and a week – when they don't introduce the baby to wider family, but simply batten down the hatches and bond as a small unit first.

When you think about the very modern discovery of the microbiome, this idea may have some extra wisdom in it. In the crucial time after the birth, when the baby's microbiome continues to be 'seeded', do we really want to be passing our baby around a large group of people? Perhaps it's better to 'keep it in the family', not just for the tranquillity of bonding, but for the sake of the microbial colony of our newborn?

Whatever you decide, it's good to plan for the first few weeks of your little one's life. Even if you are determined to spring back into action and visit Waitrose, the gym and the office on day two, you might find that the reality is a little more... hectic. Here are my tips for creating a tranquil babymoon, easing you into family life as gently as possible:

- Cook and freeze nutritious meals in advance. Pick meals that appeal to you and don't sweat about calories or iron content and the like too much: your body will recover from birth and make milk just fine and you don't need anything special. Just food that you enjoy, that nurtures you and makes you feel good.
- Don't eat your whole freezer stash in the first couple of weeks! It will be so helpful when your little one stops sleeping all the time and chopping veg one-handed is just too much for your sleep-deprived mind to handle.
- Ask friends or family who want to help to gift you a casserole or a lasagne. Even ready meals will be most welcome on tough days when there is nothing in the fridge.
- Book a grocery delivery to turn up on day two or three, with lots of easy grazing food like cold meats, cheeses, nuts, fruit, pittas, houmous, cakes and anything else you think you would like to indulge in!

- Stock up on essentials before the birth, like loo roll and toiletries. Ask for help – don't be a martyr and hit the shops if you can text a friend and get them to pick something up for you, or get it delivered. Take every single offer of help you get.
- Even if you plan to have a 'schedule' for your baby, don't bother with that for the first few weeks. Listen to their cues, feed on demand, and sleep when they sleep. Unplug from technology as much as you can. Let yourself well and truly off the hook.
- Don't plan any outings for the first couple of weeks and try not to get out of your dressing-gown if possible. Wearing a dressing-gown makes your unavailability for real-life tasks abundantly clear, both to yourself and others.
- Enjoy this precious time. Little moments when you, your partner and your baby are curled up in bed together, a shaft of sunshine coming through the curtains and casting a warm glow on your baby's peachy sleeping face – these are the moments you will remember all your life, no matter how tired or overwhelmed you may feel at the time.

All about... Breastfeeding

Like all the other choices covered in this book, breastfeeding is not for everyone. If there are physical or emotional reasons, or life circumstances, that make you feel that breastfeeding is absolutely definitely not for you, then feel free to skip this section – no bother. However, if you're planning to breastfeed or maybe a bit unsure or undecided, then grab a cuppa and read on...

Like a positive birth experience, successful breastfeeding isn't just in the lap of the gods – there is a lot you can do to 'maximise your chances'. Experts suggest that the number of women who actually have a physical barrier to breastfeeding at all is very low – exact figures are hard to establish, but it's certainly less than 5 per cent. But in spite of this, many women set out with intentions to breastfeed – in the UK around 80 per cent feed at birth – but by six weeks only around 20 per cent of babies are exclusively breastfed. Only 1 per cent of babies in England are exclusively breastfed until six months old, in spite of NHS and WHO recommendations that they should be.

If you want to breastfeed, you need to ask two questions: why is the breastfeeding drop-off rate so high? And what can I do to avoid becoming part of that statistic?

The reasons why women 'give up' breastfeeding vary – sometimes it's just too intense, and some women, particularly those with a history of abuse, can find it too physically and emotionally draining. Often there are cultural reasons – women have not seen any other women breastfeeding, and they may feel anxious about feeding in public or even in front of close family. Then there's the fact that most women are completely unprepared for motherhood itself and are shocked by the way their cute little newborn can take on what seems like vampire qualities during growth spurts or even just... all the time. The boobie can become a soft target: 'Surely it would be easier/they would sleep better/I would get my life back if I bottle fed?' Bad news: nope. Motherhood – the breast or bottle version – is tough, and it's here to stay.

Above all of these reasons, however, the worst Boobie Trap of all is simply Bad Advice. As you know – being pregnant – you're already fair game to be told you shouldn't be buying blue cheese by strangers in the supermarket queue. Unfortunately the birth of your baby doesn't herald the end to this you've been hoping for – quite the contrary. Prepare yourself for a few decades of further scrutiny.

It's interesting to bear in mind the way that your parents chose to feed and how this has influenced both them, and of course you! (You were there, you know!) Ask them about your own feeding story and bear in mind that, even if you were breastfed, some of the elements that we now know help breastfeeding to work – like skin-to-skin contact after birth or feeding on demand – might seem quite shocking to previous generations. Knowing this will help you to feel more confident if you get any unsupportive comments like 'You're not feeding that baby again, are you?!'

Remember also that the health professionals you come into contact with just after birth and in the first few tough weeks will also have their own feeding stories and possible prejudices. Not all health professionals have had breastfeeding training, not all health professionals have breastfed their own children and – here's a shock – not all health professionals know what they're talking about. As with birth, do not place blind faith in anyone with a name badge; do your own homework, and seek solid, evidence-based advice and support.

Get wise too to the long history of formula feeding in our culture – and always take into account just how much money would be lost by those formula companies if breastfeeding rates were improved even slightly. Formula marketing is subtle, it's clever, and above all, it doesn't want you to breastfeed. Raise your antennae a bit and watch out for free samples and subtle advertising (Follow-on milk is a totally unnecessary product invented specifically to get around the tight controls on formula ads, for example.) For more on this good books are *Why The Politics of Breastfeeding Matter* by Gabrielle Palmer, or *Breastfeeding Uncovered* by Dr Amy Brown.

The best advice I can give you about breastfeeding actually applies to the whole of parenting: 'Remember, it's just a phase'. If you can get through the first few tough weeks, breastfeeding will get easier as your baby settles into patterns and you begin to dance rather than stumble and fumble. You may find that the benefits to you and your baby go far beyond simple nutrition, as nursing your little one brings very special times of closeness and nurture that you will cherish forever.

Breastfeeding FAQs

How can I prepare to breastfeed? Give me some homework!

Feeding a baby is quite literally monkey see monkey do – in a well-known story, a gorilla in a zoo, who had been born in captivity, was struggling to feed her newborn. Keepers asked breastfeeding mothers to nurse their babies in view of her enclosure and – guess what – Gorilla Mum started to get the hang of it. In our modern world, most of us are like that gorilla – we've literally never seen anyone breastfeed. So, even while you are pregnant, try to address this. If you don't know anyone who breastfeeds, watch some films online. Good resources are:

* Breastfeeding expert Dr Jack Newman's site **breastfeedinginc.ca**
* Teach Me How to Breastfeed Rap: **youtu.be/SZ3QO-7h4YA**
* Film of 'Laid Back Breastfeeding' at **biologicalnurturing.com**

I really want to spend, spend, spend in the baby shop. What do I need for breastfeeding?

The bad news is – not much. The good news is – this leaves you spare cash for cute baby clothes and big-eyed teddies. Basically, all you need to breastfeed is a pair of boobs and a baby. Some people find lanolin cream helpful for sore nipples, while others swear by simply applying a few drops of breastmilk and leaving their nipples to air. Some people – but not all – are leaky and need breastpads. Muslins are a godsend however you choose to feed. Slings can be helpful, but you might like to wait till after you've had the baby so you can try before you buy.

I also recommend investing in a few page turning novels to make sitting still more interesting. An insulated mug to keep your cuppa hot while you faff about. Oh, and one of those claw things for grabbing stuff that's out of reach when you're trapped under a boobmaniac. Now that would be money well spent.

Right – I've done the birth thing. How do I get started with the boob thing?

The best possible way to initiate breastfeeding is very simple: skin-to-skin contact. Hold baby naked against your naked chest immediately or as soon as possible after birth and for as long as possible in the hours and days that follow. Initiate skin-to-skin frequently in the first days and weeks – it's great for bonding and it's the first thing you should try if breastfeeding is not going well.

Breastfeeding + skin-to-skin = PRONURTURANCE
Researchers have coined a NEW word for a very OLD activity! This magic combination REDUCES your risk of postpartum haemorrhage, SOOTHES both mum and baby, and BOOSTS oxytocin. The research concluded: 'If pronurturance was a drug it would be aggressively marketed internationally.'

OK – there's a brand new person on my chest in their birthday suit, what next?

The best thing you can do now is nothing. There's a tendency for the hour after birth to be filled with texting and status updates, and for mums to be up and dressed 24 hours later. This interrupts a really crucial time when you literally need to be somewhere dimly lit and quiet, gazing at your baby and breathing in the beautiful smell of the top of their head. Not only is this time irretrievably special, it will help you to produce all the right hormones for milk-making, and begin to learn your baby's feeding cues. Your baby will naturally gravitate towards your nipple. Trust them to get on with it and don't try too hard. Sleep with your baby near to you too.

What's colostrum?

Colostrum is the almost invisible magic potion that your boobs produce in the first two to three days. If you do see it you'll notice it's deep yellow in colour and it's packed full of antibodies, nutrients and vitamins – for these reasons many call it 'liquid gold', or 'baby's first immunisation'. After colostrum, your milk comes in, and you may notice your baby is unsettled or crying more on the evening of day three. She is telling you to have her on the breast more because she needs your body to start making lots of wonderful milk to meet her increasing needs.

How do I know if baby is getting enough milk?

This can be a common worry, but the answer is simple: check their nappy. In the early days, think one wet and one dirty nappy for each day of life. Once your milk comes in (around day three or four), poo should be mustard yellow and runny and may come several times a day – but a good guide is a minimum of two poos the size of a £2 coin every 24 hours. Wet nappies will increase to five or six in 24 hours. You can expect your baby to lose some weight in the first three days – about 5 per cent of their birth weight. After that most babies gain 5 to 7oz per week.

How often should I feed my baby?

You can't feed a baby too often. Watch their cues and if in doubt, bring them to the breast. Avoid trying to get your baby into a feeding routine, especially in the first few weeks, as this could affect your supply. The more baby nurses, the more milk you will make. Keep on boobin'!

What is a 'good latch' and why do people keep going on about it?

Basically, the 'latch' – the way that your baby is positioned at your breast and how they are taking your nipple into their mouth – can make a great difference to how well they are feeding. If they are not 'latched on' well they may not be getting milk out effectively, and since milk production works on a supply/demand basis, this can mean your supply does not establish well. A simple guide is 'nose to nipple' – this means that the baby has to tip their head back slightly to get a good mouthful of breast, with the nipple going towards the top and back of baby's mouth. It's probably easier to actually see it rather than read about it, so it's great to spend time watching babies 'getting it right' online (the Jack Newman site is great for this). If you think your baby is not latched on well, break the seal by sliding a finger gently in to release their mouth from the breast – and try again. If you are in ongoing pain from feeding, or your baby is not gaining weight, get expert advice on your latch, and also consider whether your baby has a tongue-tie.

Tongue-tie, what's that?!

Tongue-tie is fairly common, with some studies suggesting it can affect up to 10 per cent of babies. Of these, it's estimated that about half will have serious feeding difficulties. The 'tie' is caused by a piece of skin under the tongue called the frenulum being too short or too tight and restricting tongue movement. This can cause the baby to have difficulty in making the 'seal' required to suckle well from breast or bottle. In some babies the tie is obvious, whereas in others, the tongue appears normal to the untrained eye.

Common signs of tongue-tie include poor weight gain or supply issues, clicking sounds when feeding, sore nipples, and greenish nappies. Specialist advice is needed, and if your baby is diagnosed with tongue-tie, a simple procedure to 'snip' the tie can transform your breastfeeding experience.

Where can I find more support?

Breastfeeding support is out there – you just need to know where to look. Words of wisdom can come from mothers who have breastfed or are breastfeeding, from local breastfeeding support groups, from breastfeeding counsellors, either in person or on helplines (for example the ABM helpline: 0300 330 5453 or La Leche League: 0845 120 2918). There are also some great online resources such as the website www.kellymom.com and many Facebook communities such as Dispelling Breastfeeding Myths, Kellymom, or LLL Breastfeeding Matters. A good rule is that the harder you are finding breastfeeding, the higher the level of support you need to seek. The highest level of support is an IBCLC (International Board Certified Lactation Consultant). Ideally all new mothers should have access to this level of support, but it is essential that you seek it out if you are struggling to breastfeed.

REMEMBER: SCALE UP!
The harder you are finding breastfeeding, the higher level of support you need to seek. If you are struggling, but you really want to breastfeed, get specialist help, and fast!

Do I have to eat and drink anything special? And what about wine?!

Many new mums worry that, if they are going to breastfeed, they will need a special diet of unusual salad items, homegrown organic lentils, and oily fish that they caught themselves with a pole and line while babywearing. This is totally false, but such rumours serve the formula companies well, making breastfeeding sound like it might be an even more expensive faff than the bottle version. In fact, research has shown that women's milk is of roughly the same composition regardless of what they eat. This is because the nutrients in breastmilk are taken from the fat stores your body laid down in pregnancy, not the Wagyu beef fillet you ate yesterday. Eat and drink as you normally do, strive (and sometimes fail) to be healthy, as you normally do. Rumours also abound that different foods will affect the baby, in particular that spicy foods, or 'gassy foods' will upset your baby and give them wind or 'reflux'. There's not much evidence for this, and although some mums report their babies respond in certain ways to certain foods, this is mainly anecdotal and varies so much from baby to baby that the main 'take away' point here is – eat what you like. And if you want to wash your broccoli curry down with a glass of red – go ahead. Breastfeeding experts are unanimously agreed that moderate drinking when nursing does not affect your baby. For more info see the link to the Breastfeeding Network factsheet in Resources.

I'm panicking and having doubts

Keeping a cool head in the early days of motherhood is harder than it sounds as you have the most precious person in the world, right there in your arms, and she is depending on you to keep her alive, right?! Scary stuff. The responsibility of breastfeeding can sometimes feel overwhelming and you might worry about how much milk your baby is getting or whether you can keep going with it at all. But, as with birth, so with breastfeeding: if there is no immediate danger to anyone's health, take a deep breath and consider your options. If you are determined to breastfeed, introducing a bottle early on could be the beginning of the end, jeopardising your milk which works on a supply and demand basis. So make sure you have explored all other avenues, especially high-level support, before you do this.

Lactation Consultant Emma Pickett gives her top tips for mums planning to breastfeed

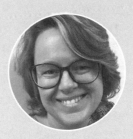

☀ **Think positive**
Believing that breastfeeding is going to work and your faith that it probably will is part of your arsenal. Those who start with, 'Well, I'm going to give it a go and just see what happens. It might not work' are missing a piece of the puzzle. There will be tough moments, almost certainly, but the truth is that the vast majority of women who really want to breastfeed, do make it work.

☀ **Do your homework**
Take some time to understand what breastfeeding does for your baby and what not breastfeeding may do. There are links to research here: **unicef.org.uk/BabyFriendly/About-Baby-Friendly/Breastfeeding-in-the-UK/Health-benefits**

☀ **Read**
Read books like *The Food of Love* by Kate Evans or *The Womanly Art of Breastfeeding* by La Leche League International. Read about other parenting choices that link with breastfeeding success. Research tells us that many mothers who breastfeed sleep in the same bed as their baby for all or at least part of the night. Have a look at **isisonline.org.uk** for information on safe sleep.

☀ **Know what's normal, or find someone who does!**
Make sure you have an understanding of the relationship between 'supply' and 'demand' in breastfeeding, what a good latch looks like and what is a normal pattern for the first few days. Problems arise when you don't realise what is normal, get help too late and struggle to find help when you need it.

※ **Write a feeding plan**
Got your birth plan? Write a feeding plan too. One sheet of
A4 with your priorities for skin-to-skin and that early feed,
phone numbers of national helplines and local support and
some key phrases to help you focus on what early latching and
positioning will look like.

※ **Find local breastfeeding specialist support**
Don't leave this until you are sitting there in a dressing-gown
with sore nipples, wondering what happened to the last couple
of days. Who offers specialist help in the hospital? Which
breastfeeding charity is active in your local area (La Leche
League, the Breastfeeding Network, ABM or NCT)? Perhaps
even go along to a group and see some breastfeeding up close
before baby comes.

※ **Get the gift of expert advice!**
If someone asks you what lovely present they can buy you – the
baby wipe warmer or the cashmere booties? – ask for a session
with a qualified lactation consultant (IBCLC). Get one round to
check your latch and positioning in the first few days. You can
find your local LC by checking **lcgb.org** listings.

※ **Get your partner and family on board**
If you really want to breastfeed you need the people around
you to understand how it works too – so share your new
knowledge with them! We don't live in a culture where we've
absorbed latching and positioning and normal breastfeeding
behaviour since we were little girls. We live in a culture where
bottle-feeding has been the norm for decades and as infants,
fewer of us were breastfed than at any time in history. This
may take a bit of work, but the things that matter usually do.

Will it always be this hard/exhausting/ boring/time-consuming?

Breastfeeding a newborn is like a crash course in meditation. Never in your whole life will you have had to sit so still for such long periods – often with your mobile phone or the remote control tantalisingly out of reach. In the first days and weeks, it will seem impossible that you can continue to live your life like this – as a feeding machine for this tiny dependent creature. But be patient, because things will improve. As you get more confident, you might learn to nurse on the move, either holding your baby or better still in a good sling. Your baby will gradually settle into a pattern and before you know it they will take longer between feeds; blink twice and they'll be sitting up and refusing point blank to eat your lovingly prepared organic lasagne. In the meantime, think of the experience as an exercise in mindfulness. Use the time to rest. Contemplate your recent birth experience, the changes in your life that motherhood will bring, and pay attention to your new emotions. Let the whole massive life-shift that's just taken place slowly settle, as you gaze at your baby and let the milk of love flow.

A quick guide to expressing, aka pumping

Women express milk for a variety of reasons, including:
- Their newborn is not taking to the breast but they want to maintain supply (often the case with premature babies, see page 238)
- They want to increase their supply
- They want to store up milk so that they can delegate feeds to dad or other relatives
- They want to keep breastfeeding after they return to work.

If you want to pump:
- Don't buy a pump – hire one until you work out which – if any – is best for you.
- Some women express by hand, but this can be labour intensive if you need to produce larger amounts or express regularly.
- Don't panic if nothing comes out. This does not mean you don't have enough milk for your baby. The process of pumping is very different to breastfeeding and many women struggle to get milk out, especially initially.

- Don't feel you 'have' to delegate feeds to dad or anyone else, if you don't want to. Breastfeeding brings a unique bond between you and your baby, and you don't have to share it if it doesn't feel right. Dads and other relatives can find other unique and special ways to share love and connect with baby.
- Unless you are pumping for your newborn because breastfeeding is not established yet, it's best to wait until about six weeks, when your supply is established and your baby has got the hang of breastfeeding, before you pump or introduce a bottle.
- Looking at a picture of your baby can help you to produce more milk when pumping – if you are separated from the baby themselves. Otherwise – look at them!
- Breastmilk should be stored in sterile containers such as plastic bottles or breastmilk bags. Milk should be labelled with the date,

Human milk for human babies?

In our culture, we are a bit phobic about human milk. We quite happily shoot dirty looks at the mum feeding her baby in the café, while calmly sipping on our latte. The irony, that most of us would be revolted by the idea of drinking breastmilk but consume a fair amount of cow booby milk without giving it a second thought, is rarely noted. So, the idea of giving your baby another woman's breastmilk might jar at first, and you might feel more comfortable with the idea of formula.

However, a growing number of women are sharing their breastmilk via Facebook groups such as Human Milk for Human Babies (see Resources). If you are unable to produce milk, or if you are ill or unable to breastfeed your baby for any other reason, donated breastmilk is another option to consider. These groups work by connecting you with a woman in your area who has breastmilk to donate. Everything works on a trust basis and no money changes hands. Once you are in touch with the group, they will give you more guidelines about the safety of donated milk. But since most of the women involved are feeding the same milk to their own babies, and are offering to help other women for free, then it seems like a great alternative to formula might just be donated breastmilk, or the milk of human kindness as I prefer to call it.

and kept in a fridge for no longer than five days. In a freezer compartment it can be stored for up to two weeks, and for up to six months in a freezer below -18 degrees.

- Breastmilk should never be microwaved. Allow to defrost or warm by leaving at room temperature and use immediately. Do not refreeze.
- Bottle-feeding of breastmilk should mimic breastfeeding. Use a slow flow teat, feed on demand and never encourage a baby to take more than they need. Generally speaking, babies will take less breastmilk than they will formula, since it is a different 'product' and fulfils them in a different way.
- The average recommended pumping time is about 15 to 20 minutes.
- If pumping becomes a way of life, there are helpful resources such as electric pumps and pumping bras that will make life easier for you.
- You can find some great information about all aspects of pumping on the website KellyMom (see Resources), including a breastmilk calculator to work out how much milk your breastfed baby might need for each session you are away from them.

Why breastfeed?

Genuine choice must be informed choice. If you're not sure that breastfeeding is for you, consider:

For baby: not breastfeeding is linked to ear infections, tooth decay, chest infections, diarrhoea and vomiting, death from gut infections in poorly and premature babies (necrotising enterocolitis), obesity later in life, lower educational attainment, and SIDS (cot death).

For you: not breastfeeding increases your risk of breast cancer, and may increase the chance of ovarian cancer. Not breastfeeding can affect your mental health and increase the risk of postnatal depression.

Benefits we can't measure

There are other benefits to breastfeeding that are harder to measure than lowered risk of health issues. Nursing brings a deep connection with your baby and is a warm, loving and nurturing act that babies find hugely comforting. Some think of breastfeeding as a 'parenting tool', a way of soothing your little one, helping them sleep, nurturing them during illness or teething, and calming emotional storms in both mother and baby.

Nursing in Public: NIP

It seems like not a week goes by without a news story about a mother who is told to 'cover up' when nursing her baby in a café, swimming pool or park. This is understandably off-putting to new mums, who may be just getting the hang of breastfeeding. Some new mothers even feel anxious about going out with their new baby, or feed in public toilets because they are so concerned that a stranger will take offence.

This is slightly strange to me because I've breastfed three children over the past eight years in every location you could imagine and never had one negative comment. In fact, the only words from strangers have been positive – most commonly older women have come up to me and said, 'I think what you're doing is wonderful'. Have I just been lucky?

I've asked other breastfeeding mothers about their experiences and the majority seem to have had similar experiences to mine. Some report the occasional 'look', but most say they have only ever had positive remarks. Some admit that the only negativity they have experienced has come from people they know – close family or even partners. The group of seasoned breastfeeders I spoke to offered the following tips for NIP:

Breastfeed in groups. While you build your confidence, find a 'breastfeeding buddy' who you can go for a coffee with – you might feel braver if you NIP with a friend the first few times. Alternatively, join your local breastfeeding group and use this as a place to practise feeding your baby in front of people you don't know so well.

Don't look for the looks. Be confident and don't look around anxiously when you are breastfeeding or seek approval in any way. You do not have to ask permission to breastfeed; the law says that you have the right to feed your baby in any location.

Wear a drapey cardigan or carry a muslin. Once you get the hang of breastfeeding you will be able to do it without exposing any more flesh than you would if you were wearing a V-neck. Your baby's head will cover your breast and nipple. However, while you are still a beginner, you might like to wear or carry something that can help you feel more confident while you are getting your baby latched on. You don't need a special 'nursing cover'; a nice drapey cardigan will do the job just fine.

Be proud to be a trailblazer. The reason we've all got such a big hang up about NIP is because we hardly ever see anybody doing it. By breastfeeding in public, you're not only doing your baby and your own health a huge favour, you're paving the way for other women to do the same. You're entitled to feed your baby anywhere you like, and if people don't like it, that's their problem, not yours.

If you can't breastfeed or you don't want to

Some people choose not to breastfeed at all, or try it and decide it is not for them. Others may be prevented from breastfeeding by life events, illness or physical issues such as mastectomy or breast surgery. Most prescription drugs are safe to take while nursing, but some are not (see the Drugs in Breastmilk Helpline in Resources). In other cases, emotional issues can be a factor. Some people who have survived sexual abuse find breastfeeding particularly difficult, for example.

No mother should ever be judged for her choices. If you can't or don't wish to breastfeed, remember:

- The next best thing to breastfeeding is not formula! The World Health Organisation sets out your choices in the following order.
  1. direct breastfeeding
  2. your own milk pumped and fed in a bottle
  3. another mother's pasteurized, screened, donated breastmilk
  4. formula milk
- If you feed formula, you can still return to breastfeeding. Many of the breastfeeding organisations in the Resources can give you advice on relactation.
- Bottle-feeding can be done in ways that mimic breastfeeding and therefore offer some, but not all, of the benefits. This is known as 'paced bottle feeding', and includes paying attention to your baby's feeding cues and feeding them in a more upright position with frequent pauses, to help prevent over-feeding. Some parents also enjoy bottle-feeding skin-to-skin. For more information search for 'paced bottle feeding', and 'UNICEF guide to bottle feeding' on the web.

All about... Postnatal Emotions

Self-care

'Self-care' is a bit of a buzzword – once you've had your baby, you might hear your health visitor, for example, telling you that you need to 'take time for self-care', or you might hear the following widely shared advice:

'If you are on a plane with your baby in an emergency situation, you will be advised to put your own oxygen mask on first, and then attend to your child.'

In other words, you can't take care of others if you yourself are struggling. Very true, but when you have a newborn baby, this is easier said than done! Tiny babies, especially if they are breastfed, really need to be with their mums most of the time, and many mums find that the feeling is mutual! You might feel like you don't want to leave your baby with someone else, and I think it's important to say that this is a normal and valid feeling, even though there is often a lot of pressure on mums to do so. Kindly relatives may suggest that you hand your baby over to them so that you can 'get some rest', or 'have some time to yourself', but if you don't feel ready for that separation, it's OK to decline.

However, as your baby gets a little bigger, it is important to do things that make you feel good. Spending time with your baby may be one of those things. For example, participating in fun activities with them like baby groups, taking them swimming, putting on music you love and dancing with them, or just having a long soak in the bath and some lovely skin-to-skin with them, can all be great, life-affirming and bonding experiences.

If you have the offer of help from someone close to you, you might also like to take time to do things that make you feel good without your baby, for example an exercise class, a coffee or glass of wine with a friend away from the house, a massage, buying yourself a treat, meditation or a long walk.

It can be difficult to make self-care a priority when you have a small baby, because, as you are about to discover, they demand a huge amount of your time and energy. But just working small moments into your routine that are 'just for you' – even if it's just a hot shower every morning by yourself – can be a vital way to stay mentally and physically healthy, and therefore better able to care for your baby.

Your post-baby body

Remember how I stood in front of the mirror when I was pregnant and thought, basically, 'Oh shit'? Well I did it again about three days after the birth. In the whirlwind of new motherhood, I hadn't really had time to catch my breath, but on day three my partner took the baby and I had a shower by myself. As I stepped out on to the bath mat, I caught a glimpse of myself. 'Oh shit', I thought. 'Oh shit, oh holy shit.'

I had never seen the body of a woman who had just had a baby before, and frankly, it was a total shock. It seems I'm not alone – remember the furore when Kate Middleton stood proudly before the photographers with her one-day-old baby George, and all the world's media could say was, 'Eh? Why has she still got a baby bump?'

So, here is the honest truth, which you may never have even considered. Once you have had your baby, your body will not return to the way it was immediately, and in fact it might be forever altered. To begin with, your tummy, where your bump used to be, will look a bit like a deflated balloon, and you may have stretch marks. Every woman is different, and while some bodies will go back to their pre-baby shape or similar fairly quickly, some will take a lot longer, and some will never be the same again. Likewise, some women will prioritise getting back into their former shape or fitness levels, while others will choose not to, and to stick with their newfound, softer form. It is up to you.

Social media is a great place to see the reality of post-baby bodies, as real women and celebrities alike often share images and feelings about their post-partum shape. The emotions often seem to be mixed – there is an acknowledgement that there is a great social pressure on women to 'go back to normal' after childbirth, and that indeed, many of us mums mourn the loss, not just of our pre-baby bodies, but of our social lives, careers, bank balances and more! But, in contrast to this, there is also an undercurrent of pride: motherhood is an incredibly special state, and you don't get to achieve it without a few war wounds, or well-earned tiger stripes.

My own relationship with my post-baby body is still evolving. After the shock of seeing my newborn mummy-bod in the mirror that day, I've had two more children, so change and upheaval is much more familiar territory for me now. I find it helps to see myself through the eyes of my kids, who find my body warm and soft and a source of great nourishment and comfort, and who never ever compare it to anyone else's body, or judge it.

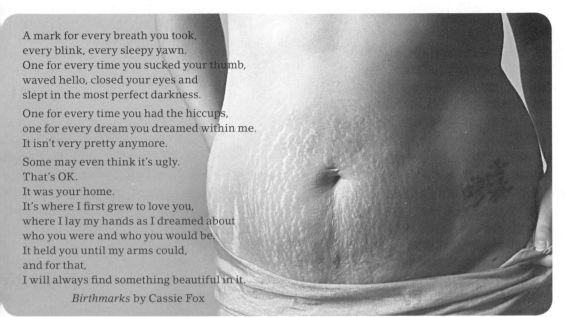

A mark for every breath you took,
every blink, every sleepy yawn.
One for every time you sucked your thumb,
waved hello, closed your eyes and
slept in the most perfect darkness.

One for every time you had the hiccups,
one for every dream you dreamed within me.
It isn't very pretty anymore.

Some may even think it's ugly.
That's OK.
It was your home.
It's where I first grew to love you,
where I lay my hands as I dreamed about
who you were and who you would be.
It held you until my arms could,
and for that,
I will always find something beautiful in it.

Birthmarks by Cassie Fox

Debriefing from birth

No matter what kind of birth you had, you may like to have some kind of 'debrief' afterwards. Having a baby is intense, and in Labour Land you don't always have a strong sense of time or even hear what is being said to you. Afterwards, you may find yourself thinking, 'What just happened?!'.

Almost every woman who has ever given birth has a strong need to talk about it. Who wouldn't?! It's a massive life event and one of the most extraordinary physical and emotional experiences a human is ever likely to have. But often, in our culture, there just isn't the time or space for these conversations. Women who want to talk about how brilliant their birth was can feel awkward and worried they will upset others who had a more difficult experience. And those who had a tough time can either raise concerns – 'Do you think you are depressed?' 'Are you bonding with your baby?' – or find the opposite happens and we are silenced: 'You'll soon forget it', 'Enjoy your healthy baby'.

No matter what kind of birth you had, if you need to talk about it, do so. Here are some suggestions for places and people that might help if you want to unpack your birth experience.

Your partner. Ideal, especially if they were there, although remember that they may also be processing the experience in their own way.

They may also have very different memories of what happened.

Positive Birth Movement. These free to attend groups always welcome new mums who want to share their birth stories – although they are not the right place to process trauma.

A doula. Even if you did not have a doula at your birth, you might find a doula in your area who will sit with you and listen to your birth story.

Your midwife. You can ask to go over your notes with your midwife and they can help you put your labour memories in a more chronological order. This may be done more formally at around six weeks after the birth at your request. This is sometimes called 'Birth Reflections' or 'Birth Afterthoughts'.

Independent Midwife. Even if you did not have an IM for your birth, you may like to obtain your notes and talk through what happened with an IM, who will be impartial but will understand the clinical side of the story. Obtaining NHS notes can cost around £50, and the IM will also charge a one-off fee for their time.

Birth trauma support. Remember, the only criteria for a traumatic birth is that it leaves a woman feeling traumatised. If this applies to you, you can contact the Birth Crisis helpline, and there are several groups on social media that offer peer to peer support, for example the Birth Trauma Association on Facebook. (See page 291 for more on birth trauma.)

Finding things tough, the baby blues, and postnatal depression

Giving birth is actually a fantastic rehearsal for the task of motherhood, although most of us don't realise this at the time. Even the best of labours can feel relentless. There are little breaks, but then another wave of intensity comes, and at times you feel like shouting, 'Stop, I want to get off!' But, unlike most things you've undertaken up to this point in your life, you have to see this through to the end – there is absolutely no get-out clause.

And then... finally... you are holding your baby, and you think, 'I've done it, it's over!' There is a short time of lying back on pillows and feeling pretty chuffed with yourself. And then the hard work really starts.

'My baby seemed so intense, wanting to feed about 15 times in 24 hours, crying a lot, and only being calm when she was carried in a sling.'

'I felt anxious, overwhelmed by the intensity of my feelings, and terrified I would do something wrong and cause her distress or harm.'

'Suddenly, being a mum brought up all kinds of really tough feelings about my own mum not really being there for me when I was little. I felt worried I would let my baby down, like she did.'

'It was all pretty quiet for the first couple of weeks, and then the colic started. Sometimes he cried so much I would just start crying with him.'

'I didn't know what I was doing and spent almost all night, every night, sat up in bed holding my baby, who I realised much later was not feeding, but happily asleep on the boob! She was content – I was beyond exhausted.'

With motherhood, as with birth, there is absolutely no let-up. I defy any woman to say she was not blind-sided by the overnight, overwhelming transformation to her life when she had her first baby. It's normal to feel this way, but while some may get a buzz from their new sense of purpose, others have mixed feelings, and around one in 10 will develop a mental health issue, most commonly adjustment disorders, anxiety, and depression.

> **"Making the decision to have a child – it is momentous. It is to decide forever to have your heart go walking around outside your body."**
> Elizabeth Stone

The baby blues

Many women experience low mood or feel tearful, often around the third or fourth day after the birth, which is usually when your milk also comes in. It's normal to feel this way and normally will only last a few hours or a few days at most. It's true that there is a lot going on with your hormones at this time, which may be the reason for your blues, but it's also a time when you will be settling back down to earth after your birth experience, and taking stock of your new situation as a 24-hour carer of an utterly dependent creature! Not easy, and totally normal to feel emotionally a bit all over the place.

Postnatal depression

For some women, however, the blue feeling may lift but then return with greater strength, or simply persist and worsen. If this happens to you, you may have postnatal depression, or PND. Like all mental health issues, there is often a stigma with postnatal depression, perhaps made worse by the fact that early motherhood is widely publicised as a time of great joy and fulfilment. For those who do not find this to be their experience, or who even have negative thoughts about the baby they are presumed by others to be doting on, it can be hard to speak out. However, the help and support is out there, so if you think you may be suffering, take heart, and read on.

Around 1 in 10 women will be affected by postnatal depression – or PND – within the first year of their baby's life. But how do you tell if you are one of them, and whether the perfectly normal emotional response to the changes that motherhood brings has shifted into something that is harder to cope with?

Some of the signs of PND might be:
- Always feeling sad or low and being unable to find the positives
- Not enjoying life, and not being interested in anything
- Feeling like you are not bonding with your baby, or interested in them (however, you can be depressed and totally in love with your baby, too!)
- Feeling isolated from others, or not wanting to make contact with others
- Thoughts that worry or upset you and are unwelcome or involuntary, for example, thoughts of harming your baby (these are sometimes called 'intrusive thoughts')

You may also feel tired a lot or have trouble sleeping, but of course this is quite common for all new mothers! Getting some rest can be very helpful to your mental health, so, if you feel your sleep deprivation is affecting your mood, try and get some support to have a few hours' sleep while your partner or other family member looks after your baby.

Who gets PND?

Anyone can get PND. If you have had any previous history of depression or other mental health issues, or have family members who have experienced depression, you may be more at risk. You may also be more likely to become depressed if you have a lack of support from friends and family, if you have issues in your relationship with your partner, or if you have gone through a difficult life event, such as a bereavement. However, you can still get PND if none of these things apply to you, and if you had a positive birth experience.

How to get help

Sometimes PND happens so gradually that it is hard to recognise in yourself, and it is your partner or other people in your life who express concern about you. If you or those close to you think you may have PND, speak to your GP or health visitor. Most health professionals are well trained in the signs of PND, and what to do to help you. If you are advised that what you are experiencing is 'just a phase', the 'baby blues' or that you should 'focus on your healthy baby', get a second opinion, or contact one of the PND charities or support networks (see Resources). Generally, the sooner you get help and support with PND, the better.

How is PND treated?

There are many ways to move forward and out of the 'long dark tunnel' of PND, including:
- Antidepressant medication
- Talking therapies like CBT, counselling, and psychotherapy
- Self-help methods such as running, resting, healthy eating, time out for an activity you enjoy, meditation and mindfulness, and more support in the home.

Birth trauma and post-traumatic stress disorder (PTSD)

Whether or not you have had what people may think of as a 'difficult birth', you may still develop PTSD, or some of the symptoms of it. Often, women who refer themselves to health professionals with some of these feelings or symptoms are told that they have PND, and given antidepressants. Unfortunately, although PND can go hand in hand with post-traumatic stress disorder (PTSD), the two are very different conditions, and antidepressants will do little or nothing to help you if you are feeling traumatised or if you have PTSD.

About PTSD

PTSD happens to women who have felt out of control during their birth experience. If you are reading this book, I very much hope that this is not the kind of birth experience you will have, and certainly, having a clear idea of the birth you want, of your rights in the birth room, and of the way you expect to be involved in decisions about your care and treated with dignity and respect, should all have a positive impact on reducing the likelihood of your beginning motherhood feeling disempowered and traumatised.

PTSD is not so much about 'what' happens to you in birth, but 'how' it happens. For example, if you had a natural birth, but were treated unkindly by a professional and repeatedly refused pain relief when you asked for it, you might develop PTSD, whereas if you had a difficult birth that ended in caesarean, but felt you were kept informed and consulted throughout, you might not develop PTSD.

There may also be some rare circumstances where traumatic events happen to you in birth that nobody can control or make easier, such as life or death situations for you and your baby.

But, to put it simply, there is no particular 'criteria' for feeling traumatised. If you feel you are traumatised from your birth, then you are. As with PND, if you think your concerns are being diminished by a healthcare provider, seek an alternative opinion, or contact some of the PTSD and birth trauma organisations in the Resources.

'Trauma is about the injury, not the event. It's like breaking a bone. I might fall down a big flight of stairs, and walk away unscathed. On the other hand, I might trip up over nothing, and break my ankle. One cannot predict this, or control it. The person who broke their ankle is not weaker or more stupid, and they cannot "pull themselves together".' Mia Scotland, psychologist

The symptoms of PTSD include:

- Being 'haunted' by memories: the persistent reliving of the event through flashbacks, nightmares and intrusive thoughts.
- Being unable to sleep or being afraid to sleep because of nightmares.
- Avoiding talking about the trauma or any situation where they might be reminded of it.
- Turning inwards, feeling lonely and isolated, detaching from your feelings.
- Feeling angry, irritable, or constantly on your guard.

How to get help

The best treatment for PTSD is psychotherapy. Speak to your GP and ask to be referred. There are also peer-to-peer networks of support such as the Birth Trauma Association Facebook group. For more see Resources.

Post-partum psychosis

Post-partum psychosis, or PPP, is a rare but serious condition that affects about 1 in every 1,000 women who give birth. It's sometimes known as puerperal psychosis or postnatal psychosis.

How do I know if I have it?

The symptoms of PPP usually start within two weeks of giving birth, but can sometimes begin later, for example when you stop breastfeeding or when your periods return. PPP usually involves a combination of hallucinations (seeing or hearing things that aren't there) or delusions (believing things that are not true). Because these hallucinations or delusions will seem very real to you, you may not realise that you are ill, and it will usually be friends or family who notice that something is wrong and seek medical help for you.

Other symptoms of PPP include feeling very elated or excited, losing touch with reality, being depressed, anxious or confused, feeling that your mind is racing, feeling paranoid, or behaving in ways that are out of character or control.

You are more likely to get PPP if:

- You have had an episode of PPP in the past
- You have another mental health condition, for example schizophrenia or bipolar disorder
- You have a relative who has experienced psychosis

If you have any of these risk factors, or have any other concerns about your postnatal mental health, talk to your midwife or doctor in your antenatal appointments. They will be able to put a care plan in place for you that means, if there are any issues following the birth of your baby, you will be able to get the help you need as soon as you need it.

How and where to get help

You or your partner or family member should talk to your GP immediately if they think you may have PPP. If they are worried you are out of hours they should call an out of hours service, and if there is any concern for your immediate wellbeing or that of your baby, they should call an ambulance.

How is PPP treated?

If you have PPP you will normally be admitted to a psychiatric unit and offered antidepressants or anti-psychotic drugs. Unfortunately there are only a few mother and baby units in the UK so, if there is not a place for you at one of these units, it is possible you may have to be separated from your baby for a short time until you are well again. If you wish to continue breastfeeding you should discuss with your care providers ways that they can support you to do this.

All about... Sleep in the first weeks and months

Sleep is so important to our emotional and physical wellbeing – but why does nobody tell our babies this?! Chances are, if this is your first baby, you've never really had any experience of being woken up several times each night – and then having to get up with the sparrow's fart just because your baby says so. It can be a real shock, and I'm afraid I can't really help much, except to say, from one mother to another – this is normal, it sucks, and it will pass.

Babies are not really built to sleep for long stretches, and they have a strong need, not just for milk, but also for love and reassurance, during the night just as much as they do during the day. For the first few days or weeks of life they live in a kind of topsy-turvy world where they don't have any sense at all of the difference between day and night, and after this, they settle into more of a rhythm and routine, quite naturally and often in spite of, rather than because of, any efforts on your part.

Nevertheless, just because they've got the hang of the day/night thing, doesn't mean your trials are over. Many babies will wake frequently for love and milk in the night for months or even years. You may be told that this is simply a 'bad habit', but I do feel that this often grossly underestimates the human need for comfort and reassurance that babies and small children have, and the great privilege that it can be to be the person who can provide it.

Privilege, schmivilege I hear you say, I just want some sleep! People resort to a wide variety of methods to try to fix their baby's sleep 'problems' (which are usually no 'problem' whatsoever for the baby!). If you feel you need to take action, I will let you and your family judge what approach is best for you. Some people cope better than others with broken sleep, and if you feel the situation is impacting on your life in major ways, for example affecting your relationship, or your physical or mental health, then do seek support.

Many parents find that simply having more realistic expectations of their baby's sleep makes them feel better. Sharing a room with your baby is also very helpful, and many mums, especially those who breastfeed, find that taking their baby into their bed allows them to get a lot more rest. If you do this, it's important to follow the guidelines for safe co-sleeping.

- Don't share a bed with your baby if you or your partner are a smoker or have consumed alcohol, or drugs (recreational or prescription)
- Make sure your mattress is firm and do not sleep with your baby on a sofa or in a chair
- Co-sleeping is safer if you are breastfeeding. Formula-fed babies sleep differently and their mothers can be less attuned to them
- Don't share a bed with a premature baby
- Don't co-sleep if you are obese
- Keep the baby away from any duvets or pillows and make sure your baby cannot fall out of bed or become trapped between the bed and the wall
- Do not sleep with your baby if you are exceptionally tired
- The safest kind of co-sleeping is planned co-sleeping. If you want to share a bed with your baby, think in advance about how you can create a sleeping environment that is safe and works for everyone

You can find some suggested reading and support for night-time parenting in the Resources. I particularly recommend the Infant

Sleep Information Service **isisonline.org.uk**, who have a wealth of evidence-based information on normal baby sleep, and some great resources for parents, including a free app.

All about... Bonding with your baby

'Bonding' and 'attachment' are buzz words when it comes to the epic task of looking after a newborn. For many people, a deep connection and bond with their baby comes naturally, but for others, it can be tougher or more complicated. A difficult birth or breastfeeding experience can have a negative impact on your ability to bond with your baby, and perhaps even more so than this, your own childhood experiences of being mothered or parented can suddenly rise up and become painful to you as you begin this new relationship with your own child.

If you are finding connecting with your baby particularly hard, it may be worth exploring your feelings around motherhood with a counsellor or therapist, or just someone you trust like your partner or a close friend. Getting to the root of your difficult emotions may help you to move forward and develop a stronger relationship with your child, thus breaking the cycle and allowing them to have the experience of being loved freely that you may not have had yourself.

'Attachment' and 'Attachment Parenting'

Psychologists and psychotherapists are largely agreed: the quality of the bond and attachment between a baby or child and their 'primary caregiver' (that's you!) lays the foundations for good mental health for the whole of the rest of their life. The idea of attachment comes from a psychologist in the 1950s called Bowlby, whose 'attachment theory' – the idea that the presence and consistency of a parent figure has a fundamental influence on human development – is a cornerstone of modern psychology. Bowlby felt that 'mothers matter', although one of his contemporaries, Donald Winnicott, was careful to clarify that it was not possible to be a 'good mother', but that 'good enough mother' is what we should all be aiming for. Phew.

In recent times some of the thinking from attachment theory has been taken on by parenting experts and evolved into a style of parenting known as Attachment Parenting (AP). AP involves integrating activities into your parenting style that promote bonding and attachment, for example babywearing, bedsharing, and rejecting

Babywearing

A decade ago, carrying your baby in a sling was considered a pretty radical step, the preserve of hippies and tribal people only. These days, thanks mainly to celebrity babywearers such as Beyoncé, Pink and Gwen Stefani – plus a few hot dads like Orlando Bloom and Brad Pitt – slings are de rigueur on the maternity shopping list. As well as being a way to look trendy when you've got sick in your hair, poo up your nails and haven't had three hours' consecutive sleep in weeks, carrying your baby in a sling has countless benefits for both you and your baby, including:

☀ **Happier babies**
Babies are often happier, cry less and nod off to sleep with ease when walked around in a sling. Many studies have found that babies who are carried cry much less than those who are not. Being in a sling mimics the gentle rocking movement of being in utero and can help your baby feel safe. They can also smell you, hear your heartbeat and your voice, and in general feel closer to the mothership than they would in a buggy. This is particularly great for premature babies (see Kangaroo Care, page 239).

☀ **Bonding**
There's nothing like a sling for giving you easy access to the top of your baby's head, the smell of which will fill you with a special kind of joy. In a sling you can talk to, stroke, and sniff your baby, and you will find they soon do the same in return. It's a very loving and snuggly environment and the benefits of this early attachment are well documented: babies who love and feel loved carry this sense of self-worth through life. Love and affection, and the responsiveness that accompany them, also help build your baby's brain by enabling them to understand and make sense of the world through the medium of you – yes, you; the one who's busy sniffing their head.

☀ Attunement

Parents who carry their babies can find it easier to tune in to their needs and notice when they are hungry, uncomfortable or unhappy. This means they can respond more quickly to their needs, which in turn leads to more confident and contented babies who know that their needs are going to be quickly met. Babies carried in slings are also more attuned to the environment around them: they are up at the level of adults and can more easily see, hear and begin to make sense of the world.

☀ Convenience

Slings are great for Getting Stuff Done. The more you get the hang of them, the more activities you'll be able to do while your baby happily nods off, breastfeeds (yes, this is possible!) or just observes carefully the minutiae of your Tesco shop. It's much easier to go for walks across the fields, or navigate train stations and airports, when your baby is in a sling. Many slings also fold small enough to fit in your bag, so you can get in the habit of never being without one. And as well as being smaller than buggies, they are also an awful lot cheaper!

For more information about the importance of babywearing, sling safety and the different types of sling, try *Why Babywearing Matters* by Rosie Knowles. In many areas sling libraries and sling consultants can give you real-life help with any questions.

other modern parenting styles that suggest we should 'train' babies and not always respond to their cries.

Much of the advice from AP experts and organisations (see Resources) is excellent, but it's important to know that, just because you may choose to put your baby to sleep in a separate room or push them in a buggy, does not mean that you will be any less bonded or attached than someone who takes the AP path. In fact, the World Health Organisation stresses the importance not of Attachment Parenting, but of 'responsive parenting'.

Responsive parenting

Responsive parenting begins at birth, or arguably even before. Many new parents will talk to their baby in utero, sing to them, and if they see or feel a kick, will interact with them and respond. In the moments after birth, new parents will soothe the cries of their newborn, blow on their face, kiss them, and offer words of love. You will see many new parents in these moments, tuning in so deeply to every little expression on their baby's face, copying the expressions in their own face, and echoing their baby's sounds with their own sounds. This is responsiveness in action.

As your relationship and bond with your baby develops, your responsiveness will continue. Neuropsychiatrist and parenting expert Dan Siegel talks about the four S's: your baby or child needs to feel 'Seen, Safe, Soothed and Secure'. By continuing to tune in to your baby, you will be able to develop a relationship built on love and affection, a relationship in which your baby knows they can rely on you to give prompt and appropriate responses to their needs.

The benefits of responsive parenting are far-reaching. Quite simply, they create a template for all of your baby's future relationships, teaching them the deep joy and security that comes from loving and being loved. Deeper than this, they teach your baby how to have this relationship with themselves: how to value, care for, listen to, respect and respond to themselves, just as you are doing for them.

Sue Gerhardt's ground-breaking book *Why Love Matters: How Affection Shapes a Baby's Brain* is a must-read for new parents. She explains how vital the first loving relationship is to a baby's neurological development, and on those days when you are desperately tired, and perhaps a little bored of baby care, I think it's so helpful to remember the importance of the work that you are doing. A game of peek-a-boo may feel repetitive, but it is helping your baby develop their sense of self. A teddy game that results in fits of giggles might wear thin for you, but your baby is being flooded with positive hormones that make them feel wonderful. A little one that cannot sleep without being cuddled may be tiring you out, but they are developing their prefrontal cortex in ways that will help them to have empathy for others. These small 'motherly' actions are great gifts with far-reaching consequences.

Conclusion

A few years ago, I gave a talk about the Positive Birth Movement and at the end, a woman from the audience came up to me to tell me what a wonderful idea she thought it was. She was in her seventies, and as she began to talk to me about her own birth experiences in the 1960s, her voice became charged with emotion. She still remembered how, after her second baby was born, she had been forced to 'rest' in hospital for a week, meaning she was kept apart from her beloved toddler, who she felt needed her at this time of transition more than ever. She had never been away from her first child, and was so overcome with guilt and anxiety at this sudden separation that she struggled to bond with her newborn. Over half a century later, her eyes filled with tears as she recalled these painful memories that had stayed with her for a lifetime.

She is not alone. Women of all ages remember their birth experiences in great detail, holding on to them forever. When we listen to them, we can learn so much about positive birth. Fundamentally, what each and every one of them tells us is that, while the birth experience itself is very important to them, it is the wider emotional details that matter even more. Women want different things from birth, just as they want different things from love, sex, career, and life itself. Many want to birth naturally, to feel that power in their body as they bring new life forward. Others want strong pain relief, or may choose to birth in theatre. But what they all have in common is the desire to feel in control, empowered, respected and listened to. They want to feel like they matter, and that the people around them understand this fully and treat them like the goddess that somewhere, deep down, they can absolutely feel that they are.

We have come a long way from the births of the 1960s and 70s, when so many women found that things were happening to them and their bodies that they did not want or agree with, but felt powerless to argue against. Now we would find it impossible to consider a woman being made to stay in hospital, separated from her family against her will. We would just say, 'Walk out! It's your right!', but back then women were more likely to do as they were told. If the doctor said you were getting an enema next, or matron said your baby was being taken away to the nursery, then that was what happened. However, it's a mistake to think this imbalance of power is completely fixed: history is a continuum, and the 1960s and 70s were not so very long ago.

If you take anything away from this book, I hope it is the knowledge that you can be the most powerful person in the birth room. You can speak up and use your voice and ask questions and say what you want and need. You can challenge decisions that don't feel right to you. I hope that the information contained in this book gives you the confidence to do this, and – in my dream scenario – to work in partnership with your care providers to get the best possible birth. Not a one-size-fits-all birth, but a tailored, unique experience that reflects who you are as a person and that you will remember forever with warmth and pride.

At the start of this book, I offered you a tandem skydive, but of course, this can only ever be virtual – it's unlikely I'll actually be there at your birth (although feel free to invite me!). And no matter who else is with you as you have your baby, birth is ultimately a solo mission – it's you and you alone who can birth this baby, just as you and you alone can be their mummy. Daunting stuff. You're certainly going to need a parachute – or maybe even a jetpack – for the giant leap of faith that bringing new life into the world and taking care of them forever requires of you. Pack it carefully, and don't forget to include as many life-saving elements as possible: a strong support network, the love of your partner and family, attention to self-care, patience, the ability to ask for help, as well as a shit-hot birth plan and the knowledge of what you really need for birth and how brilliant it can be that you've hopefully found in this book. Above all, have courage. You can do it.

Acknowledgements

Like a baby, a book would not come into being without the involvement of a whole lineage of people who may never come to know the power of their influence or even meet the small act of creation that they somehow helped to bring to life.

So many people have been part of the writing of this book, either by their influence on my thinking or by giving me their wisdom direct.

I could never name all of the people who have supported, informed and cheered me on via social media, but I am nevertheless grateful to every single one of them, particularly those who took time to describe their birth experiences in detail, some of whom (but by no means all!) are featured in Chapter 2.

I'd also like to thank Abigail Blackburn, who believed in me as a writer and helped my confidence, ideas and skills grow as my editor at BestDaily.

I'd like to thank the following people for their expertise and support: Amanda Burleigh, Beverley Beech, Carol Bartle, Caroline Hastie, Catherine Williams, Ciara Curran, Clare Goggin, Cristen Pascucci, Donna Booth, Dr Alison Barrett, Dr Amali Lokugamage, Dr Andrew Mayers, Dr Florence Wilcock, Dr Liz Martindale, Dr Maria Gloria Dominguez-Bello, Dr Raja Gangopadhyay, Dr Richard Porter, Hannah Tizard, Heidi Eldridge, Jenny Clarke, Julia Clark, Katheryn Gallagher, Kicki Hansard, Kylie Pattnaik, Leigh Kendall, Maddie McMahon, Mars Lord, Mary Newburn, Mia Scotland, Michele Ball, Natalie Corden, Natalie Meddings, Professor Lesley Page, Rebecca Dekker, Rebecca Schiller, Rosie Goode, Shawn Walker, Sheena Byrom, Sophie Fletcher, Toni Harman, Michelle Quashie, Virginia Howes, Erika Thompson and Zoe Clark-Coates.

For their stories: Arianwen Harris, Beki Kemp, Emma Bateman, Erika Townend, Felicity Jeffreys, Frederique Rattue, Gemma Cash, Georgina Graham, Gerri Wolfe, Hannah Bragg, Hannah O'Sullivan, Hannah Roe, Hayley Goleniowska, Hannah Winbolt Lewis, Jody

Deacon-Viney, Kate Hewitt, Louisa Aldridge, Natalie Dybisz, Sarah Berryman, Shalome Doran, Michelle Wyatt and Tricia Murray.

For their influence:
Ina May Gaskin, Jana Studelska, Janet Balaskas, Karin Ladefoged Walters, Kate Woods, Michel Odent and Sheila Kitzinger.

For bringing the book to life:
Martin Wagner, Maria Pinter, Rebecca Winfield, Emily Furniss, Zoë Hutton, Susan Last and Kate Evans.

I'd like to hug the following midwives:
Tara Windmill-Robson, Caroline Baddiley and Chrissy Hustler.

Extra special thanks and love to my mum Pauline Hill.

And finally a big chaotic group hug to my three wonderful children Bess, Ursula and Albie and my partner George Litchfield, who are my absolute world.

Resources

Antenatal Classes and Groups

NCT **nct.org.uk**

Active Birth **activebirthcentre.com**

Positive Birth Movement **positivebirthmovement.org**

Daisy Birthing **thedaisyfoundation.com**

Birthlight **birthlight.co.uk**

YogaBirth **yogabirth.org**

YogaBellies **yogabellies.co.uk**

Birth Support

Doula UK **doula.org.uk**

IMUK **imuk.org.uk**

DONA International **dona.org**

Birth Trauma

Birth Trauma Association **birthtraumaassociation.org.uk**

Great peer to peer support in their Facebook group 'Birth Trauma Association'

Birth Trauma Trust **birthtraumatrust.org**

Facebook group: 3rd & 4th Degree Tears (or severe/episiotomy) Support

Breastfeeding Support and Information

Kellymom **kellymom.com**

Association of Breastfeeding Mothers **abm.me.uk**
ABM Helpline: 0300 330 5453

La Leche League **laleche.org.uk**

LLL Helpline: 0345 120 2918

Breastfeeding Network **breastfeedingnetwork.org.uk**

National Breastfeeding Helpline 0300 100 0212

Drugs in Breastmilk Helpline 0844 412 4665

NCT **nct.org.uk**

Lactation Consultants UK **lcgb.org**

International Lactation Consultant Association **ilca.org**

Jack Newman **breastfeedinginc.ca**

Nancy Mohrbacher **nancymohrbacher.com**

Breastfeeding and Alcohol Factsheet from the Breastfeeding Network **breastfeedingnetwork.org.uk/wp-content/dibm/alcohol.pdf**

Human Milk for Human Babies **hm4hb.net**

Facebook pages:

The Milk Meg, The Analytical Armadillo, KellyMom, Dispelling
   Breastfeeding Myths, LLL Breastfeeding Matters

Books:

The Womanly Art of Breastfeeding by La Leche League International,
   Pinter & Martin, 2010

Dr. Jack Newman's Guide to Breastfeeding by Jack Newman, Pinter &
   Martin, 2014

Ina May's Guide to Breastfeeding, Ina May Gaskin, Pinter & Martin, 2009

Why Breastfeeding Matters by Charlotte Young, Pinter & Martin, 2016

Breastfeeding Uncovered by Amy Brown, Pinter & Martin, 2016

Food of Love, The: Your Formula for Successful Breastfeeding by Kate
   Evans, Myriad, 2008

Caesarean Birth

Caesarean Birth **caesarean.org.uk**

Facebook pages: Caesarean in Focus, General Anesthetic Caesarean
   Mamas

YouTube: The Natural Caesarean – A Woman Centred Technique

Complications

Pregnancy Complications and Symptom Checker **tommys.org**

Preterm Prelabour Rupture Of Membranes (PPROM) **little-heartbeats.org.uk**

Group B Strep **gbss.org.uk**

High BMI **bigbirthas.co.uk** (also on Facebook)

Down's Syndrome: Downs Syndrome Association **downs-syndrome.org.uk** and Downs Side Up **downssideup.com**

Edwards and Patau's Syndrome: **soft.org.uk** and **emilysstar.co.uk**

Early days of parenting

Infant Sleep Information Source **isisonline.org.uk**

The Wonder Weeks **thewonderweeks.com**

Attachment Parenting **attachmentparenting.co.uk**

Gentle Parenting **gentleparenting.co.uk**

Books:

Sweet Sleep: Nighttime and Naptime Strategies for the Breastfeeding Family by La Leche League International, Pinter & Martin, 2014

The Gentle Sleep Book by Sarah Ockwell-Smith, Piatkus, 2015

Why Your Baby's Sleep Matters by Sarah Ockwell-Smith, Pinter & Martin, 2016

Why Love Matters: How Affection Shapes a Baby's Brain, Sue Gerhardt, Routledge, 2014

What Mothers Do, especially when it looks like nothing, Naomi Stadlen, Piatkus, 2005

Our babies, ourselves, how biology and culture shape the way we parent. Meredith F. Small, Doubleday, 1999

Kiss Me!: How to Raise Your Children with Love by Carlos González, Pinter & Martin, 2012

Evidence

Which? Birth Choice **which.co.uk/birth-choice**
Easy to use site with info and stats on all UK maternity units

BioMed Central **bmcpregnancychildbirth.biomedcentral.com**
Open access, peer-reviewed journal on all aspects of pregnancy and childbirth

Cochrane Reviews **cochranelibrary.com**
The highest standard in evidence-based healthcare resources

Royal College of Obstetricians and Gynacologists **rcog.org.uk/ guidelines**
Great search facility for their Green Top guidelines or others such as NICE Guidelines

NICE Guidelines **nice.org.uk**
May be easiest to search via the RCOG site, see above

The American College of Obstetricians and Gynaecologists (ACOG) **acog.org/Resources-And-Publications/Practice-Bulletins-List**

Society of Obstetricians and Gynaecologists of Canada (SOGC) **jogc. com/clinical-practice-guidelines**

Evidence Based Birth **evidencebasedbirth.com**
US based researcher Rebecca Dekker gives a really accessible overview of the evidence relating to many of the major birth choices and dilemmas.

Fathers & Birth Partners

Dean Beaumont's site **daddynatal.co.uk**

Mark Harris's site **birthing4blokes.com**

Books:

The Expectant Dad's Handbook: All you need to know about pregnancy, birth and beyond by Dean Beaumont Vermilion, 2013

Men, Love & Birth by Mark Harris, Pinter & Martin, 2015

The Father's Home Birth Handbook by Leah Hazard, Pinter & Martin, 2011

Home Birth

Homebirth Reference Site **homebirth.org.uk**

Facebook pages: Home Birth UK, Home Birth Chat UK

Books:
The Homebirth Handbook by Annie Francis, Vermilion, 2016

Home Birth by Nicky Wesson, Pinter & Martin, 2006

Home Birth: Stories to Inspire and Inform edited by Abigail Cairns, Lonely Scribe, 2006

Books for children:
Our Water Baby by Amy Maclean and Jan Nesbit, The Good Birth Company, 2006

Hello Baby by Jenni Overend and Julie Vivas, Frances Lincoln, 2009

Hypnobirthing

Katherine Graves **kghypnobirthing.com**

Wise Hippo **thewisehippo.com**

Mindful Mama **mindfulmamma.co.uk**

Marie Mongan **us.hypnobirthing.com**

Natal Hypnotherapy **natalhypnotherapy.co.uk**

Books:

Mindful Hypnobirthing by Sophie Fletcher, Vermilion, 2014

Why Hypnobirthing Matters by Katrina Berry, Pinter & Martin, 2015

Mental health

Action on Post Partum Psychosis **app-network.org**

Association for Postnatal Illness **apni.org**

Pre and postnatal depression advice and support **pandasfoundation. org.uk**

Support for those with maternal OCD **maternalocd.org**

pndandme.co.uk
  hosts of #PNDHour on Twitter

Book:

Why Perinatal Depression Matters by Mia Scotland, Pinter & Martin, 2015

Microbiome

Filmmakers and writers Toni Harman and Alex Wakeford's site: **microbirth.com**

Book: *The Microbiome Effect* by Toni Harman and Alex Wakeford, Pinter & Martin, 2016

Miscarriage and Stillbirth

Saying Goodbye **sayinggoodbye.org**

Sands **uk-sands.org**

4 Louis **4louis.co.uk**

Optimal Positioning

Spinning Babies **spinningbabies.com**

Dr Eliot Berlin's film on Breech Heads Up **informedpregnancy.com/heads-up**

Breech Birthing **breechbirthing.com**

Facebook pages: Unlocking Birth, Breech Birth UK

Placenta Encapsulation

IPEN **placentanetwork.com**

Pregnancy Information

Mama Academy **mamaacademy.org.uk**
  Baby movements and more

Pelvic Partnership **pelvicpartnership.org.uk**
  Info on pelvic girdle pain

Pregnancy Sickness Support **pregnancysicknesssupport.org.uk**
Support for sickness and hyperemesis gravidarum

Disabled Parent **disabledparent.org.uk**
Info and support for disabled parents

Mummy's Star mummysstar.org
For women and families affected by cancer in pregnancy and beyond

Tell Me A Good Birth Story **tellmeagoodbirthstory.com**
Find a 'birth buddy' tailor-matched to you

NHS Choices **nhs.uk/Conditions/pregnancy-and-baby**
Pregnancy information and advice

Orgasmic birth **orgasmicbirth.com**

Midwife Thinking **midwifethinking.com**
Highly informative blog from Australian midwife Rachel Reed

Evidence Based Birth **evidencebasedbirth.com**
US-based researched Rebecca Dekker looks at the evidence on hot topics

Which? Birth Choice **which.co.uk/birth-choice**

Apps:

Digital Doula *Postnatal support, doula style*

Ask the Midwife *Instant advice from a midwife*

Baby buddy *Personal baby buddy for pregnancy and the first six months*

Wonder Weeks *Track your baby's psychological development &
understand fussy phases*

Mind the Bump *Mindfulness and meditation for pregnancy and early
parenthood*

Clue *Period and fertility tracker*

Podcasts:

The Birth Hour, Rockstar Birth, Sprogcast

Facebook pages:

Birth Without Fear, Belly Belly, The Positive Birth Movement,
Optimal Cord Clamping #waitforwhite, Ten Month Mamas (*Group for
those who want to explore alternative options to induction for post-dates
pregnancy*)

Books:

Birthing from Within: An Extraordinary Guide to Childbirth Preparation, Pam England and Rob Horowitz, Partera Press, 1998

Ina May's Guide to Childbirth, Ina May Gaskin, Vermilion, 2008

Becoming Us: 8 steps to Grow a Family that Thrives, Elly Taylor, Three Turtles Press, 2014

Water Birth: Stories to Inspire and Inform, edited by Milli Hill, Lonely Scribe, 2014

Bump: How to make, grow and birth a baby by Kate Evans, Myriad, 2014

Premature babies

kangaroomothercare.com (especially their book, Hold Your Prem)

Bliss **bliss.org.uk**
For premature or sick babies

YouTube film: Procedure in the NICU Uppsala, University Hospital Sweden

Pre-eclampsia

action-on-pre-eclampsia.org.uk

preeclampsia.org

Rights in pregnancy and birth

Birthrights **birthrights.org.uk**
Promoting respect for human rights in UK birth

HRIC **humanrightsinchildbirth.org**
Promoting human rights in birth globally

Maternity Action **maternityaction.org.uk**
Employment and working rights for UK pregnant people and parents

AIMS **aims.org.uk**
Promoting normal birth, rights and choice. Helpline & support.

AIMS Ireland **aimsireland.ie**
Promoting choices and rights in Ireland

Improving Birth **improvingbirth.org**
  Advocating for evidence based birth in the USA

White Ribbon Alliance **whiteribbonalliance.org**
  Demanding the right for a safe birth globally. See their Respectful
  Maternity Care Charter

Book:

Why Human Rights in Childbirth Matter by Rebecca Schiller, Pinter &
  Martin, 2016

Twins

Twins and Multiple Births Association **tamba.org.uk**

VBAC

VBAC Support Group UK on Facebook

VBAC stories: lotsofvba3cstories.blogspot.co.uk and **vbac.co.uk**

Special Scars **specialscars.org**
  Support for women with atypical incisions and unusual scars

Book:

Vaginal Birth After Caesarean: The VBAC Handbook, Helen Churchill
  and Wendy Savage, Pinter & Martin, 2010

Visual Birth Plan

You can download the visual birth plan icons from chapter 6 of this
book from the Pinter & Martin website:

pinterandmartin.com/vbp

Index